Praise for *Just Listen for the Thud*

"Evocative and captivating, *Just Listen for the Thud* gives us permission—even encourages us—to laugh at the roadblocks and detours in our journey of caring for others. Caregiving is an imperfect art that is frequently frustrating, but can be fulfilling if viewed with humor instead of dread. Maggie Pike captures the stories of these caregivers in an honest light we can all relate to."

Teresa Lewis Pisano, RN
Care Manager
ALS Association Golden West Chapter

"Beautifully written! With lightheartedness—even fun—*Just Listen for the Thud* gives us a glimpse of the complexities of caregiving along with the opportunity to balance the joys and frustrations of the special caregiving relationship. As a caregiver, I appreciate Maggie Pike's welcome reminder that we are not alone. I have come away with a fresh, new perspective that I can bring to my work with patients and share with their family caregivers."

Carrie McCann, RN, BSN
Senior Oncology Research Nurse Clinician
Masonic Cancer Center, University of Minnesota

"I am really impressed with Maggie Pike's approach to the storytelling in this book. The personalized chapters are engaging, touching without being maudlin. She has done a really good job of capturing each couple and humanizing each situation. This is great reading, intriguing and thought-provoking for anyone, but especially for those in a caregiving relationship."

Denny Dressman
Member of the Denver Press Club Hall of Fame and author of seven books

"Maggie Pike has an ability to tell people's stories from the heart. It was a pleasure to read these vignettes of others' caregiving journeys, and a reminder to take a moment to find the time to laugh! My husband has SPMS (secondary progressive multiple sclerosis) and before he became chair-bound, and then bed-bound, we had our own share of falls. I will say, sometimes all you *can* do is laugh!"

Rebecca Martens
Well Spouse Association

"Maggie Pike has used the intriguing approach of narrative to impressive effect. Her heartfelt portrayals leave no doubt that the roles of patient and caregiver are equally hard. The use of storytelling as a medium to educate, support, and (most importantly) normalize the fear that comes with either is powerful. We can learn a great deal about laughter, grace, and change from those who were courageous enough to share their stories with us."

Justin Collins, LCSW
Social worker for senior care and former hospice social worker

"These stories are wonderfully touching and humorous, but there's also a spiritual dimension to them. With Maggie Pike's accounts comes the appreciation of the gift of humor to accept how imperfect we all are, and to enable us to make the best of any situation in which we find ourselves. That is a good lesson for all of us, but even more powerful for caregivers."

Andy Drance, M.Ap.Th.
Retired hospital and hospice chaplain

JUST
LISTEN
FOR THE
THUD

Humorous & Intimate Stories from Caregivers

∽∾⌣∾⌣

Maggie Pike

Willow Creek Publications, LLC

Printed in the United States of America
First Printing, 2016

ISBN: 978-0-9964611-2-2

Willow Creek Publications, LLC

www.maggiemccannpike.com

TABLE OF CONTENTS

Laughter is Solace 9
Just Listen for the Thud 14

PART 1: LEARNING

ACCEPTING WHAT IS

Annette and Mike 21
"This is our life. This is how it's going to be."

Barb and Phil 26
"We had to redefine our fairy tale."

Sonja and Ken 29
"It got to where entertainment was a visit to the store for more
supplies to help us out."

Germaine and Willie 34
"I had to change the color of my lens."

Barbara and Jerry 41
"Hard work doesn't have to mean being miserable."

Pat and Bob 46
"Life is good. It really is."

CARING FOR SELF

Deri and Beaver 53
"Any time spent rejuvenating oneself ultimately results in more
quality time to spend with the patient."

JoAnn and Fred 59
"Travel seemed like the best way to keep us both interested in
life."

Callae and Lee 65
"People assumed I needed to get away. That's not what I wanted at all."

Helenn and Joe 70
"Doing for someone else was far healthier than closing myself off from meeting people."

RECEIVING HELP

Carolyn and Dave 77
"They say God doesn't give us more than we can handle. Well, he gave me a turkey platter, put a cow on it, and thought I could carry it all!"

Del and June 83
"Seeing her assigned to the care of others enlarged the hole in my heart."

Pam and William 88
"Our first rule was no self-pity. Instead, trust and obey."

Fran and Virginia 94
"Promise me you'll put me into a nursing home when you can't take care of me any longer."

Ken and Audrey 99
"This disease wasn't going to put us away. But we needed support."

LETTING GO

Daniel and Stephanie 107
"Please don't let it get too bad. Please."

Andy and Carol 113
"We love you enough to let you go."

Ruth and Jim 119
"Our life was full of serendipity."

PART 2: LAUGHING

Falling Free 127
Daniel and Joe

Ado in Honolulu 129
Carolyn and Dave

The Last Word 131
Andy and Carol

The Potato Dance 133
Callae and Lee

Limbo Like Me 134
Del and June

Cruisin' 136
Barb and Phil

Sass 138
Annette and Mike

Mission Accomplished 140
Barbara and Jerry

Road Trip Feat 143
Fran and Virginia

Cuttin' Loose 145
Helenn and Joe

Dance Therapy 147
JoAnn and Fred

Honestly, the Things a Caregiver Will Do 149
Germaine and Willie

Rising Above the "If Onlys" 152
Ken and Audrey

Dealing with Delusions 154
Pam and William

Euphemisms and Threats 156
Pat and Bob

Keeping Life Fascinating 157
Ruth and Jim

Chocolate Cake Feast 159
JoAnn and Fred

Chivalry Lost 161
Sonja and Ken

Coffee Trials 163
Andy and Carol

An Athlete and a Gentleman 164
Barb and Phil

Carolyn at the Bat 166
Carolyn and Dave

Proper Church Wear 168
Fran and Virginia

Man Cave 169
Germaine and Willie

Drive-Thru Service 171
Helenn and Joe

Clicker Capers 174
JoAnn and Fred

In Your Face, PSP 175
Ken and Audrey

Taking Turns 177
Pam and William

And the Oscar for Best Supporting Actress 178
Pat and Bob

Ticket to Freedom 180
Ruth and Jim

The Doorbell 182
JoAnn and Fred

Dancing Love Letters 184
Sonja and Ken

31 Choices 186
Annette and Mike

Escape Artist 188
Barb and Phil

Two Bucks 189
Deri, Callae, and Lee

Wedding Vows 191
Carolyn and Dave

Ace 194
Del and June

Packed to the Gills 196
Fran and Virginia

Putting Out the Flames 198
Germaine and Willie

Wrong Joe, Right Joe 200
Helenn and Joe

Hardly Injured. 203
JoAnn and Fred

Fudgsicles to the Rescue 205
Annette and Mike

Parkinson's Great Symphony 207
Barb and Phil

Noise, Glorious Noise. 209
Annette and Mike

Taming Mr. Handyman. 210
Germaine and Willie

Close Encounters Where the Deer and the Antelope Play 213
Barb and Phil

The Noble Cause of Preserving Dignity 215
Annette and Mike

Listen for the Thud and Watch for the Thug. 217
Helenn and Joe

Healing From Loss 219
Sonja and Ken

APPENDIX

Definitions of Terms 223
Tips for Caregivers 227
What is Helpful, What is Not 237

Acknowledgements 241

For JoAnn Holland

It was your dream to honor your fellow caregivers by bringing their narratives to print. Your heart of gold dwells at the core of this book.

Laughter is Solace

I'm waiting in the hallway outside Bernice's apartment. The musty smell of sickness seeps from the jagged crack of light at the base of the door. I've been through dozens of first meetings in my role as hospice volunteer, and I can't help but wonder what our time will be like, this woman in end-stage heart disease and myself. Every person, every visit brings surprises.

No answer. I knock again, more forcefully.

The door finally opens, and a woman of eighty, clad in pajamas wrinkled and stained, her hair in disarray, a yucca plant of a hairdo, pushes her walker to the side. "It takes me a while to get to the door," she scolds.

Bernice. Her rebuke takes me aback, but it's nothing personal. She doesn't feel well, for heaven's sake.

Like all hospice caregivers, I'm constantly discerning how I'll respond to the patient in that moment. Showing compassion is essential, always. Lending my shoulder as she rails at the injustice of her condition might be appropriate at times. Listening to fears, hopes, regrets—yes. Sitting quietly next to him while he rests. I move with my patient. You never know.

But this day, with this woman, in this moment, I follow my intuition: I'll have to get Bernice to laugh.

Seems almost irreverent, I know.

I learned this lesson about laughter from my dear neighbor Mary. Terminal colon cancer had prompted my visits, and during my times with her I did what I thought I should: I assumed a compassionate demeanor; asked her each time how she was feeling, what she was thinking, how she was managing her symptoms.

One day, Mary interrupted me. "I don't want to always talk about this darn illness." Pointing to the glass door to her balcony, smudged from fingers trying to get out, my friend gestured to the sunny sky waiting to welcome her into its embrace and pleaded, "Tell me what's going on out there."

From that moment on, lighthearted was the tone of our visits.

As Bernice's hospice volunteer, I'm there to simply keep her company. But from her initial greeting, my intuition tells me that, in her dark space, Bernice craves lightness. She seeks cheer.

She longs to feel that, somehow, life still holds goodness.

She yearns for solace. And laughter is part of the solace.

Yes, I know just what to do during my visit with Bernice. We will laugh.

Bernice leads me into the kitchen, shuffling with the help of her walker, the labored sound of her slippers grating against the floor like sandpaper. She wastes not a moment before explaining that this is an exceptionally bad day for her. Her pale, drawn face and dull eyes are testament to her suffering. "I feel so sick today. I just want to go back to bed," she says. "You know, sometimes I have to tell people, even my family, that this is not a good time to visit."

Bless her heart, Bernice is doing everything she can, short of kicking me out, to let me know she isn't so sure she wants or needs a volunteer to come visiting. It was her son and her hospice nurse who'd encouraged her to accept the visits.

I choose to ignore her hints. I know too much about the power of laughter in healing the spirit to withhold it from this dear lady in her final weeks. I won't stay long.

Bernice and I get to talking—and we don't stop for two hours. She covers her career, her sweethearts, her husbands, her children, her crazy neighbor, the gaffes we all make, the follies of human nature. With each topic, our faces match each other's in buoyant mirth. We're skydivers at terminal velocity, no longer accelerating toward the ground, but pushed upward by the forceful wind of humor that we can't escape. Nor do we want to.

In that two-hour span, a startling transformation occurs. Bernice's face is animated, her eyes bright, her skin now glistening and eggplant smooth as her cheeks lift in laughter. The visage before me is stunning. For this moment, Bernice's life has shifted from listless to lively.

What anyone who has cared for a gravely ill person knows for sure is that our care receivers are very much alive, with the same basic human needs they've always had. The need for humor is a crucial one. True, terminal illness is not a laughing matter. But in our worry and grief, it's all too easy to let our days turn gray. It's in our power to bring light into the journey, and laughter can salve the soul unlike anything else.

Besides, humor holds a bonus: it heals the heart and improves the quality of life for the patient—and the caregiver, too. It's hard stuff, this tending to the sick. The reality is that the disease does not belong only to the ailing; it's the caregiver's illness as well. So the question hangs in a speech bubble above the caregiver's head: *What can I do today that will make this better for both of us?* We have the opportunity to make a decision— daily—to open the door to sunshine rather than get used to the somber in our lives. We are not required to be morose.

We can laugh.

This is a book about family caregivers. The eighteen spouses and children I interviewed shared a common challenge: a fatal degenerative neurological disease. Progressive supranuclear palsy (PSP), multiple system atrophy (MSA), and corticobasal degeneration (CBD)—like the equally debilitating but better known Lou Gehrig's disease (ALS) and Parkinson's disease—are among the most challenging situations a caregiver could ever face.

But this book offers solace to those who face *any* disease that transforms an ordinary person into a caregiver, a loved one into a need-driven patient.

This is a not a book about multisyllabic maladies that are mouthfuls to pronounce—though the maladies are there. Nor is it a manual on how to one-two-three take care of a sick loved one—though the how-to is woven into the narratives.

This is, first and foremost, a book about people. People who are nurturing relationships—not just with others, but with themselves, too.

It's about the intimacy that grows between two people in the context of caregiving, a closeness that might not occur in any other situation.

It's about living the vow "in sickness and in health, till death do us part."

It's about the personal growth he experiences when thrust into a role he had never imagined for his life script.

It's about loving herself—and the other—enough to take good care of her own health and to honor friends and family by accepting their offers of help.

It's about acceptance of what is, and the freedom therein.

These are narratives about love and commitment and learning and trial and conquest. Most of all, they're testaments to the potency of laughter.

The powerhouse practice that can heal the spirit.

The key to survival.

When it comes to tending to the requirements of the seriously ill, the demands are universal, as are the healthiest ways of handling the challenges. No situation trumps another. Every life-altering illness requires immense dedication from the caregiver. Some caregivers may say they never even thought about it, that it's just what you do when you love someone. Others report they might have been overwhelmed had they known what was coming, but the changes come on slowly enough that they simply handle them and make the necessary adjustments along the way.

But for many caregivers, there is a moment when they know they have to make an internal shift or they won't survive.

It's a moment of surrender.

Not in the sense of accepting defeat, as in war. Surrender for these caregivers is a package of attitudes that has brought peace to their situations. They have given up old patterns of thinking and embraced a new outlook.

Surrender is recognizing that this new life is simply another stage of living.

It's relinquishing any illusion of power over the disease and instead walking—boldly or timidly—into the reality of it.

It's seizing the opportunity to know and be known by the other in ever richer ways.

Rising above the messiness of illness and seeing the goodness of life.

Finding new ways to be content.

Giving up the "victim" mindset.

Surrender means accepting a future without a loved one, understanding that while grieving is necessary, living a full life is still possible.

And in their surrender, they have learned to laugh.

Indeed, every one of the families in this book eventually learned that surrender meant allowing the solace of humor into their lives.

Maggie Pike

Just Listen for the Thud

Light shimmers on trembling autumn leaves as the wind ushers in a change that will eclipse the sun. Inside, protected from the coming tempest, the room is quaking with laughter in the face of a different kind of storm.

Newcomers giggle nervously. *Can I laugh? Should I laugh?*

More confident laughter erupts from those who have learned they'd better, lest the disease they face every day consume them.

Ruth is talking.

"... and there we were, another fall, both of us this time. I mean, Jim's a hundred pounds heavier than I am. So down we went. Our butts were stuck in the wastebasket, and our four legs were sticking out like cinnamon sticks in a bowl of chocolate mousse."

Thunderous laughter.

These are caregivers in a support group—spouses, partners, children, and siblings committed to sharing the journey of their loved ones who have life-threatening illnesses. It's the one place they can laugh. For now, they're cradled in the womb of people who understand.

"It's weird how we can laugh," says Daniel. "The first time my wife fell, I was terrified. I ran like crazy to help her, and my heart was pounding. I condemned myself for letting it happen. But after six or seven years, you know how often they fall. You just take care of it."

Another gentleman pipes in. "Yeah, falling *is* going to happen—many times—if we let them be independent." Voices buzz in agreement.

Finally, JoAnn speaks. "I've learned to just listen for the thud. And then I go pick him up." The room erupts again.

Adds Annette: "I just can't be everywhere at every moment. I finally decided that I don't have to panic and run with every fall. I've learned to recognize a head-banger from a thud."

Maggie Pike

Everyone gets it. They've been there.

The discussion that follows is lighthearted bantering about the types of thuds each has experienced in caregiving.

There's the dropping-the-remote thud; the falling-out-of-a-chair thud; the leaving-for-vacation thud (when you must figure out a way to go anyway); and the squishy thud, which means she or he has missed the handgrips in the shower.

More serious is the fall-between-the-toilet-and-the-sink thud. Get him out of there. Stat. If he's like Dave, who broke the tank lid in five pieces with his fall, do as his wife Carolyn did and learn, on the job, how to reseat a toilet.

Possibly most common is the answer-the-door thud. It usually occurs when a solicitor ignores the sign on the door and rings or knocks anyway. And he just *has* to get up and open the door. On the way he slips and falls, and you come home from walking the dog only to find him sprawled on the floor. Maybe even with a broken hip. That's serious, of course. Regardless, it's scary. And guilt-inducing. But as anyone who has seen this happen will tell you, having to witness the falls— and their aftermath—is the risk that comes with replacing "hovering" with empowering.

Perhaps the most charming is the sensual thud. When accommodating each other, one discovers that the other's lack of flexibility has become something of a hazard. They roll off the bed together, producing a thud that is lengthy and flat. No need to worry; both are somewhat anesthetized.

And finally, there's the thud of the heart, the one that stays inside, heard only by the caregiver as he watches the one he loves fight valiantly against a cruelty that neither one of them could have imagined—or ever asked for.

"You have to laugh," says Pat, a seasoned caregiver. "If you can't see the light side, you'll never get through this illness. And it's important to find other laughers. What I appreciate about the support group is that we provide levity for each other in the face of overwhelming challenge."

You are about to enter into the sacred space of caregiving families, first through their stories, and then through a series of anecdotes that reflect their humorous and touching responses to the question they hear most often:

"How do you do it?"

How? They learn and they laugh.

A playful "Just listen for the thud" is merely the first piece of advice they offer to anyone in a caregiver's role. But there's more. Listen in.

PART 1
LEARNING

Accepting What Is

Annette and Mike

"This is our life. This is how it's going to be."

It was two a.m. when the Fudgsicle call came, the ringing of the bell from Mike's room intruding in Annette's delicious dream. She turned over, hoping to finish it, but it had disappeared. She climbed out of bed—not reluctantly, for she did this every night—and shuffled to the kitchen where the stash of frozen treats filled a good portion of the freezer. Fudgsicles were the one thing she could not do without while caring for her husband. Once his body fluids were replenished and his mouth no longer dry, he would go right back to sleep. She kept the lights off, trying her best to stay in her twilight state so she, too, could fall asleep as soon as she crawled back into bed.

Such were the rituals that were part and parcel of Annette's world ever since PSP, progressive supranuclear palsy, invaded the couple's life. Those, along with taking up the scatter rugs, improvising a maze of bars in the bathroom to help Mike get safely from one place to the next, and padding the brick hearth, sharp table corners, and walls that got bumped by his power chair. In essence, padding the entire house. "This is just the course of life. You're born, you live, you die," Annette philosophized.

"And you learn to laugh," she added. "You laugh, or you don't make it."

But PSP was far from a laughing matter the day they received the diagnosis. In fact, it was the darkest moment of their lives. The doctor had explained that progressive supranuclear palsy was parkinsonism, a term used to describe one of a number of degenerative neurological diseases with symptoms similar to those of Parkinson's disease, yet with distinct origin, nature, and clinical course. In fact, PSP, along with two other diseases with similar symptoms, multiple system atrophy (MSA) and corticobasal degeneration (CBD), often confounded doctors in their attempt at an accurate diagnosis. Over time, slow movement, stiffness, and problems with balance, as well as trouble talking, sleeping, chewing, and swallowing would overcome Mike with increasing severity. Unique to PSP would be the inability to aim his eyes properly, especially in the downward direction. Annette could also expect personality changes that would likely include diminished interest in pleasurable activities, and frustration in not being able to express himself, resulting in irritability. Tragically, there was no treatment and no cure for Mike's condition. And the disease was extremely rare. *Wow,* Annette had thought, *if only we could be so lucky with lottery tickets.* She had rejected the "why me" victim response, knowing Mike's wellbeing—and her survival—depended on it.

Now, back to sleep, Annette thought after delivering the sweet, frozen comfort to her husband. But she wasn't able to reenter her tranquil slumber. Feelings of tenderness toward Mike filled her as memories appeared and flitted away like fireflies. More than twenty years earlier, after she had changed careers from nurse to medical-specialist flight attendant, she was working international flights with "nothing more than champagne and an oxygen tank as medical supplies," she reminisced. She had no idea the man in the next-to-the-last row—a heady petroleum engineer who'd retired as vice president of his company, a widower on his way to Alaska to go fishing with his brother—was eyeing her. And she would have been flabbergasted if she'd known what he was thinking: *That's the woman I'm going to marry.*

Six weeks later, Mike, who had cared for his wife, Shirley, through her long illness, who shared Annette's Catholic faith, prayed often, and held a devotion to Our Lady of Perpetual Help, got down on his knees, diamond in hand, and assured Annette, "God gave you to me because I stayed with Shirley till the end."

Annette chuckled as she recalled the reception that followed their wedding at her church in Seattle. It was a cake-and-coffee celebration— although it was almost just a coffee celebration, thanks to a delivery person's failure to see the "Put cake on table" note on the door. Thinking no one was home, he took the cake back to the bakery. Fortunately, he returned later, just in time for the reveling guests to appease their hunger with carrot cake. The following day, Annette and Mike began married life on their honeymoon in Santa Fe, New Mexico.

But after many happy, active years, Annette found herself in the role of Mike's caregiver. She could hear him clearing his throat across the dark bedroom. *The Fudgsicle will quiet him in a moment,* she told herself. As she rested her head on her pillow, she thought back to the time she'd taken Mike to see a throat doctor, not just because he was clearing his throat all the time, but because he was choking on his food way too often. Surprisingly, when the physician stuck a camera down Mike's throat, Mike didn't even flinch: his gag reflex was greatly diminished. The doctor could see Mike's vocal cords buckling, and he discovered that one of the cords was paralyzed.

Like so many life-threatening diseases, Mike's was not easy to diagnose, especially in its early stages. In his case, several odd symptoms signaled something was wrong, but his doctor simply took care of each indicator as it cropped up, sometimes referring him to a specific specialist.

Eight years earlier, for example, he suddenly couldn't hear out of his right ear. Then just as suddenly, his hearing returned—for one day. Then, gone again. A year to the day later, he went deaf in his left ear as well. His world was completely silent.

But then, miraculously, cochlear implants appeared on the scene. The worse of his two ears received the gift of twenty-two contacts, wires, and magnets—enough bells and whistles to warrant a special card to show TSA agents at the airport—and his other ear was equipped with a hearing aid that afforded him a forty percent hearing capacity.

The next symptom involved his speech—it came out either too fast or too slow, and his words were slurred. The doctor thought it was hearing related.

And then his motion wasn't right. The initial diagnosis of a stroke soon changed to something even more disturbing once the neurologist and movement specialist added their expertise. It wasn't long before Annette and Mike learned what a rare and complex condition Mike had.

Degenerative.

Miserable.

"Join a support group," urged the doctor.

Fortunately for Annette, Mike's symptoms came on slowly enough, and multiple misdiagnoses gave them enough hope for a cure that she didn't feel overwhelmed during the first few years of his illness. But the final diagnosis, along with their growing knowledge of the devastating nature of PSP, changed everything. There was no cure. Suffering was inevitable. Death was certain.

After a strong dose of inner struggle, the couple finally arrived at acceptance: since they couldn't change their situation, they would choose to change their attitude.

"This is our life," they decided. "This is how it's going to be."

"And I'll tell you," added Annette, "I wouldn't have missed those last four years of caring for Mike for anything. An intimacy developed between us in the context of caregiving that was an absolute gift."

Though a devoted caregiver, Annette was cautious not to ignore her own needs. She made use of aides and care centers. She even took a trip or two, leaving Mike with professional caregivers. As it turned out, Mike enjoyed the attention he got from his helpers—and they were equally charmed by him.

By the time Mike entered hospice, he had twice received the Anointing of the Sick, the Catholic sacrament that invites spiritual and physical strength during a life-threatening illness. Still on their minds, though, was the ominous former name of the sacrament—Extreme Unction, or the last rites—because in earlier times it was administered just prior to death. But apparently Mike still had some living to do because he didn't die after either anointing. They had joked that it was going to take both Annette and Shirley, Mike's late wife, one on each side, to carry him to his final heavenly destination.

The biggest challenge for the pair was concentrating on the positive, laughing at the humorous, and shooing away all thoughts negative or depressing. "Through Mike's disease, I learned to lighten up," said Annette.

She paused to stir her coffee.

"And to laugh. You have to be able to laugh." Of course, Mike's muscles wouldn't allow him to laugh, but Annette knew he shared her sense of humor in the face of darkness.

Mike eventually surrendered to the disease, the tyrant they and their doctors had thought was PSP. But Annette had fulfilled Mike's request to have an autopsy performed, and when the report came back, she was shocked and bewildered. Mike hadn't suffered and died from PSP after all—corticobasal degeneration had taken his life. And sprinkled into the report were additional sinister conditions, like argyrophilic grain disease (AGD) and dementia with Lewy bodies.

How could that be? None of those terms had ever come up in the course of his illness.

That autopsy report was Annette's difficult lesson in the challenges doctors face in trying to correctly diagnose these degenerative diseases of the nervous system, many of which have nearly identical symptoms. The fact is, since there is no cure for PSP, MSA, or CBD, the treatment is the same: take care of each symptom as well as possible to make the patient more comfortable. Annette was consoled knowing Mike had received the best care given his condition.

Mike had raged against the dying of the light in perfect Dylan Thomas fashion, but as he exited this world, Annette was right there, bringing him comfort. His deceased wife, Shirley, took his hand and led him into the next life.

Just as they'd joked, Mike's two loves got him to his final resting place.

Barb and Phil

"We had to redefine our fairy tale."

"I know this may sound unbelievable, but Phil and I really did live a fairy-tale life," said Barb. The blond, fit former college coach and athletic director looked down for a moment, remembering the time before multiple system atrophy invaded their lives. She tried to find a positive in their new way of life. "We're really fortunate that Phil has responded favorably to medications."

Quality time for Barb and Phil had always revolved around three things: travel, sports, and time with their two children. The two Pennsylvanians met in their late twenties, he immersed in his family's furniture business, she, in volleyball, basketball, lacrosse, field hockey, and anything else that post-Title IX college women played. They met at a tennis party and held to love for the next four decades. The robust couple allowed nothing to interfere with their devotion to skiing, biking, tennis, and each other.

But a family ski trip one year brought some mystery into their tale. Phil kept falling on the slopes, on runs that normally posed no challenge to him at all. His balance was off—most likely due to the powder—so he simply adjusted his technique, making larger turns. Every single day. He went back to the condo at the end of each day feeling sluggish—most likely because of all the extra effort he exerted negotiating those turns. And, most likely, because of the high altitude.

Most likely.

Phil's slower-moving demeanor followed him back home, but an outsider might not have noticed a difference. He and Barb kept up their active lifestyle, and when he had to slow down, there was always a logical reason. He hadn't slept well the night before. He'd already exerted himself at the gym. He was hungry. There was always an explanation.

A return trip the following summer to the majestic Rockies excited the couple. But one day while hiking in Vail, the story's villain made its appearance. A good deal of the trek found Phil sitting down often to regain his strength. Barb watched helplessly as his climbing turned to clambering, then to slogging. She felt a surge of panic. This time she could find no excuse. Something was drastically wrong with her husband.

Phil's symptoms pointed to a number of different conditions, so starting with his primary care physician, he ran along the track of specialists, passing over brain tumor, Parkinson's, and a few other possibilities before finally landing on the official diagnosis of MSA, multiple system atrophy.

Atrophy.

For two fervent athletes whose lives revolved around movement, that word rocked their world like no other.

Their first question was, how will this condition affect our lives?

Their next, how long do we have?

A second opinion, an internet search, and a specialist in movement disorders provided the answers. "Phil can live anywhere from three to ten more years with MSA," said the specialist. "I would suggest you get your affairs in order and do everything you want to do."

So they did. Phil's first step was to close the furniture business.

And for the next four years, Barb and Phil played. They crossed the country on trip after trip, spent winters in Florida, and encouraged their children to follow their dreams as well. They flatly refused their daughter, for example, when she said she wanted to give up her travel abroad opportunities to be there for her parents. Their response was the same when their son offered to turn down the three job offers he'd received in Colorado and instead return to Pennsylvania, where he could use his new Doctor of Physical Therapy degree to help his father: "Absolutely not." The firmness in Barb's voice reverberated across the miles. "Dad and I are living our lives to the fullest, and you should, too."

As a result, both children ended up in Colorado, and that's where Phil and Barb joined them when Phil's health started worsening and "the bad two years" began.

This is it, thought Barb. *This is the decline they warned us about.*

Phil started aggressive treatment right away with a highly recommended movement specialist in Denver. Before long, Phil was improving in every category of every test. He was looking stronger, feeling better about himself, and radiating a more positive attitude. Colorado was good to Phil and Barb. Not only were they surrounded by their two children, both of whom were living where they wanted to live and doing what they wanted to do, and not only was it sunny almost all the time, but the treatment afforded the couple a reprieve from the progressively devastating symptoms of Phil's illness.

Barb and Phil learned to laugh early on. They had to, they'll say. The reality was that in addition to crushing challenges, being caregiver and care-receiver presented them with countless funny stories of their foibles, tales that flow rich and thick like a trailing ermine cloak. The pair could spend hours recounting the ways they stared illness in the face and went on with life. They knew the choice was theirs. They could smother themselves in regret that their fairy tale was over. Or they could do exactly what they did: seize the time they had. Play like children plopped down in Disneyland. Make each day the best it could possibly be. Savor the sweetness of each other and of their children. Embrace every step of the journey, the trying and the tender, the daunting and the delightful.

And laugh. Always laugh.

In so doing, they were able to write a new fairy tale.

Sonja and Ken

"It got to where entertainment was a visit to the store for more supplies to help us out."

When a hot date meant a leisurely stroll down the colorful aisles of Babies R Us, Sonja pushing Ken in his wheelchair, the couple knew they were in a different universe. Their mission was well defined that day. They needed a two-way room monitor, maybe even one with a camera, specifically one that didn't have buttons to push. Sonja would just leave it on at all times. That way, she could hear Ken when she was working around the house. And more importantly, she could catch him at the first sound of covers crinkling, and get to him before he sat up so they would avoid the dreaded thud.

Ken was in the clutches of progressive supranuclear palsy, PSP. Gone were the days of the couple's carefree travels to Hawaii, San Francisco, and other exciting cities; Ken preferred to be at home. Things were different now. For one thing, he made it known he wasn't about to wear any of those adult diapers, so Sonja had grown accustomed to spreading plastic carpet protector on the floor around him for those times when he get couldn't get to the bathroom fast enough. She could hardly take a roll of that stuff to public places.

So the couple provided their own entertainment at home.

They started each day the same way. Sonja would get Ken up and dressed and then they'd walk a couple of laps around the house for exercise. The two leather easy chairs in the living room awaited them, one a manly brown, the other, a delicate beige. But before they took their places for the day, Ken would reach out and embrace his love. He would hold her for a long, long time. Not just that day, but every day, and not just in the morning, but again in the evening. "That intimate connection each day was so important to us," said Sonja. "It made us feel like we weren't alone."

Sonja and Ken were at once lighthearted and tender with each other. Ken, who had always been in tune with Sonja's needs, continued to help her. Before meals, he made sure the strips of shelving material, sticky and woven in texture, were under his dishes so they wouldn't slide while he was eating. Or when she was changing his bed pad, he would grab the rail to make himself lighter so his petite wife wouldn't have to work so hard. He helped her out, too, when she guided him with his gait belt, working hard to steady himself as he walked. "He was the same sweet person as he had always been. He did everything he could to make my life as a caregiver easier, just as I was trying to make his life easier," said Sonja.

One day, as Sonja and Ken were sitting in their favorite chairs watching funny movies, flames flickering and crackling in the fireplace behind them, Sonja's mind drifted back over the path of their life together.

They had met through trade shows, she a sales promotion coordinator from Ohio, he a sales manager for a different company in Chicago. But they didn't date until five years later. Sonja was drawn to Ken in so many ways. His most obvious quality was his kindness. The product of Catholic schools, he was active in his church, and while in college, he had worked as head counselor of a school for children with special needs. By the time they wed, Sonja knew firsthand that Ken was the embodiment of goodness.

"We were meant for each other," said the diminutive brunette. "With the same temperament and similar backgrounds, we got along so well. Marriage wasn't hard work for us." She paused to look at his picture on the mantle. "I realize more than ever how lucky I was. Our life together was just beautiful."

Sonja summed up her thoughts about her tall, handsome husband. "Ken's life was really about making people happy."

He was also athletic. Not only did he love biking, but he was always up for trekking with Sonja, his even more rigorous hiking partner. Her reverie led to the year the couple went to visit Ken's son, who had recently built a house on top of a mountain. The group decided to take a walk through the woods. Ken started out enthusiastically, but after a while his pace slowed, and he complained of being tired. His balance was a little off, too, but once Sonja stomped down the foliage to make the path easier, he was okay. Sonja couldn't resist teasing him about old age creeping up on him, and with that, no one thought another thing about it.

Fast forward five years. Ken and Sonja were sitting in the doctor's office awaiting a diagnosis for some unusual symptoms. His walk had gotten slower, his balance, more unsure. But what concerned Sonja even more was the vacant look in his eyes, his appearance of daydreaming. The doctor faced the couple with a grim expression. "I'm sorry to have to deliver this news," he said. "Ken's symptoms all point to Parkinson's disease, and he appears to be in the early stages of Alzheimer's."

Any shock was overshadowed by Sonja's doubt. Ken didn't fit the profile of Parkinson's that she'd read about in her research. He exhibited only minor shaking, and Alzheimer's? No, his memory was good. Clearly, they had a lot to learn. But as the couple turned to leave, Sonja had one more question.

"Doctor, we're making plans to go to Italy. Is Ken okay to go?"

The doctor looked at his patient for a moment and nodded. "Yes, just listen to his body and go at his pace," he advised Sonja. He stood up from his chair to escort them out. "But I would suggest you purchase travel insurance," he added.

Despite his diagnosis, Ken continued to maintain an active life, and Sonja kept up her service as a nanny several hours a week. They decided to go ahead and finalize plans for their trip to Italy.

The day of their departure approached, and the couple were growing excited. They would be leaving on Wednesday, so they spent Sunday attending to the final details. As they fell into bed that night, they could feel their dream vacation in their bones.

Suddenly, in the middle of the night, Sonja woke to a loud thud. She ripped off her blankets and sped to the bathroom. No one was there. "Where are you, love?" she hollered in a panic. No sound. Then a quiet voice made its way up to her. "I'm on the stairs." When she looked at the landing to her right, Sonja saw exactly what had happened. Instead of turning to the left to get to the bathroom, Ken had turned right, which sent him careening down the ten steps to the landing. Sonja was terrified. She turned the light on and saw her husband crumpled on the stairs. Thankfully, no blood was apparent, and other than a sore back, he assured her he was okay.

The next day, Sonja left the house for her nanny job. She loved the family she worked for, and spending time with their little girl always left her feeling uplifted. She wouldn't be gone long—just four hours that day—and Ken would be busy with his final medical checkup in preparation for their big trip.

Out of the blue, Sonja's cell phone rang. Her heart fluttered when she heard the words of the nurse. "Sonja," she said, "Ken didn't show up for his doctor's appointment. I tried to call him, but there was no answer."

Sonja got right on the phone and called Ken herself. This time he answered. But his words were bizarre. "Talk hard," he said. And then again, "Talk hard." Sonja called a neighbor to go check on him while she made arrangements to leave her work. When she got home, Ken was speaking normally. He recognized her and could name the people in the pictures around the house; nothing seemed amiss. Nevertheless, Sonja drove him to the hospital.

The news was not good: Ken's tumble down the stairs had caused a blood clot in his head. From there, things happened fast. Brain surgery, five weeks in the hospital, and three more months of rehabilitation replaced the trains, trails, and trattorias of Italy. And according to the movement disorder doctor, this was just the beginning. "You're not planning on taking him home, are you? He's not going to be the same man he was before."

Ken appeared to be asleep when the doctor spoke, but if he heard the dire warning, he defied the prediction. As it turned out, Ken lived quite productively until the last couple of months of his life. "He was still intelligent, even if it took him a little longer to process," said Sonja.

But Ken's disease had its heartbreaks, without a doubt. As upbeat as Sonja tried to remain, it was wrenching to see her husband's abilities grow more and more limited. Eventually, he couldn't speak or swallow, nor could he see or stand up. In fact, she had to listen to more than one thud when he forgot he couldn't stand and his muscles gave way. "His brain was still working, but he just couldn't look down," she explained.

Because of Sonja's nagging doubts about the Parkinson's-Alzheimer's diagnosis, she became more aggressive in seeking an accurate diagnosis that fit Ken's symptoms. After much effort, she was able to get an appointment with a highly reputed movement disorder specialist. "I can tell you Ken doesn't have Parkinson's, nor does he have Alzheimer's," said the doctor. "He has a rare, incurable disease called progressive supranuclear palsy. Life expectancy is about six to eight years, but I would say Ken is probably midway into the disease."

Ken and Sonja felt the thud in their hearts. Incurable. Getting worse. Only four more years together, at most. The haunting prognosis followed them out of the doctor's office. Armed with new information about PSP, and dispirited by the challenges ahead, Sonja nevertheless felt relieved that at least they knew what they were dealing with.

Over the next few days, Sonja cried inside when she heard her husband lament, "It's like being in a box." As she knew, his mind was alive, but it was locked inside. It broke her heart to see how poor the quality of his life, how difficult his physical challenges. But while Ken's needs would continue to be challenging for her, she never questioned her commitment to care for him until the end. In keeping her promise to him, Sonja sought compassionate help in their home: she called hospice.

Throughout Ken's illness, the couple had grown so in tune with each other that they moved together in seemingly effortless ways. So when the hospice team arrived at their house and observed Ken's condition, they immediately declared he wasn't ready for hospice. Sonja knew how badly he was faring, but it was hard to convince the team that Ken's seeming wellbeing had to do with the teamwork they'd worked so hard to achieve. She did, however, convince hospice to admit him on a three-month trial.

Sadly, Ken's life expectancy diminished rapidly, and instead of four years, he lived only three months after his diagnosis. Just before the end of his hospice trial period, Ken escaped from the trap of his PSP box.

A flutter of cards and letters brought comfort to Sonja in the aftermath of Ken's death. Visits from his hospice team formed a bridge of solace, connecting those last months to her uncertain future. One-by-one they came, the entire hospice team, reassuring her with the words: "We've never seen such love between two people."

Still, as she fingered each picture of her handsome husband, she longed for another one of those hot dates, even to Babies R Us.

Germaine and Willie

"I had to change the color of my lens."

"I always tell people I was married to the perfect man," says Germaine, her eyes twinkling with mischief. "And Willie was half of that man. The other half was my first husband, John. I loved them both, yet they were so different from each other. I got the best of each of them, so together they made a perfect husband."

Germaine and Willie became a unit when Germaine's son invited his mother and his coworker, Willie, to a singles' dance. Both had been widowed after nearly forty years of marriage, but while the outgoing Germaine was ready to kick up her heels, Willie was dragging his feet. "Grumpy" might better describe him that night. It was only later that Willie admitted he thought Germaine's son was trying to push them together, and he wanted nothing to do with it. But once *he* was in charge of the decision, Willie recognized the charm that was Germaine, and they began dating.

Marriage followed. "I always thought it was a compliment to our first spouses that we would want to enter into our second marriage," says Germaine. Their combined eleven children got to witness a slightly unorthodox wedding: the couple held their reception before they actually tied the knot. Because they were eager to get their honeymoon started, they didn't want to waste time chitchatting after their nuptials, so the reception came first. It wasn't until the next day that they actually got married. An hour after the wedding ceremony, the couple boarded the plane for their three-week honeymoon in San Francisco and Hawaii.

"Willie had a great personality and was always so thoughtful," reflects Germaine. Throughout their twenty-five years together, he would bring her flowers and candy, and often planned surprise getaways. And while they were both working, the two shared household chores equally.

Then one year, they decided to buy a Toyota RV—a used one,

34

just in case they didn't really take to life on the road. But they took to it, all right. For two weeks at a time, year after year, the couple would take their places in the cab and explore every part of the United States, the blur of trees changing color and shape with the seasons and locales as they whizzed past. As often as they could, they opted for the back roads, where café food was home cooked, invitations to "just stay here" were aplenty, and people were warm and gracious. Their kind of folks. Which is not to say they always played it safe. One year, they found themselves lost in the shadowy part of a big city after a wrong turn, their wheels squealing as they raced to escape the people who were taunting them.

Just four years into their marriage, Willie began to develop health problems. Mysteriously, finger infections, sinus infections, prostate infections, facial cysts, and plantar warts converged on him like a flock of foraging birds. His triple diagnosis—infection of the nerve endings, spinal stenosis, and osteopenia in the thoracic spine—required steroid injections and pain medication, along with physical therapy.

This didn't slow the couple down much, though. They weren't going to let a few inconvenient aches and pains interfere with their fun.

Fifteen years later, back pain caught up with Willie. Surgery on his lumbar spine promised to fix him right up again, but less than two months after spinal surgery, Willie wasn't walking well. That was when Germaine heard the first thud. Her husband suffered a hairline crack on his tailbone as a result. "Willie, you're always in a hurry," Germaine chided. "If you would just slow down, you wouldn't fall so often." But Willie continued to fall. Often.

A year after his operation, Willie was still receiving pain medication, steroid injections, and physical therapy, and now occupational therapy and water therapy were part of his weekly regimen. For his constant pain, the doctor tried a nerve stimulation system used by people with Parkinson's disease. No improvement.

Soon a new, even more troubling symptom appeared. Willie's voice was failing him. A diagnosis of vocal cord atrophy sent him to a speech therapist, but his barrage of ailments was baffling to his doctors. Even though his spinal surgery had been deemed successful, Willie's balance, gait, and speech were problematic after the operation.

The following year, Willie met with a neurologist for his failing motor skills and his headaches. By now he had dropped thirty-five pounds. The neurologist prescribed Sinemet, the dopamine-replacement medication for Parkinson's patients, but it brought no improvement. Two weeks later, suspecting Willie might have a vitamin B-12 deficiency rather than Parkinson's disease, the doctor ordered a test. Willie's B-12 level was normal. The only logical conclusion at that point was that Willie had parkinsonism, a symptom complex, rather than Parkinson's disease itself. Willie's next stop was to the office of a movement specialist, an expert in Parkinson's, progressive supranuclear palsy, and multiple system atrophy.

Meanwhile, Germaine suffered a setback herself. Ten days after a total right shoulder replacement, she tripped over her dog, causing her to dislocate her other shoulder. That injury required a second operation on the original shoulder; the surgeon completely redid the right shoulder replacement.

Germaine and Willie's home was beginning to resemble a comedy of errors—not only was the two-slinged Germaine caring for her husband, but for her mother, Ruby, as well. Her hundred-year-old mother. For a while, the threesome had to combine their respective limited capabilities to create a whole caregiver. Germaine needed arms, Willie needed legs— or at least a guardian angel to slow him down when he walked. Ruby, despite her age, was the most self-sufficient of all during that time.

While Germaine did not resent her role as caregiver, she secretly looked forward to the day she and Willie could resume their previously carefree life.

But it wasn't long before Willie's movement specialist delivered the dreaded diagnosis: Willie had probable progressive supranuclear palsy, PSP, verifiable only by autopsy.

The scenario was not going to get better.

His falls became more frequent; whenever he started walking, his legs would lock, causing him to tumble. One of his therapists advised him to stop and look at his toes, study them for a moment, and then proceed. Well, it worked like a charm—except that once he mastered the strategy, he often left Germaine in the dust, she trying her best to keep up with her roadrunner husband.

But soon, Willie was falling three to five times a day. One summer afternoon as the sun sat on its mid-sky throne and thrust its ninety-degree scepter rays onto Germaine and Willie's yard, Germaine came home to the back door open. She gasped. She'd given Willie strict orders not to go outside until she returned from the store, but he was gone. She sprinted outside and stopped suddenly on the porch. There was Willie, lying in the rock garden below, every blistering stone searing his skin through his clothing. Frustration filled the normally patient Germaine like a surge of bubbles in a shaken soda can. She had to find a way to protect Willie from his falls, but none of his bruising and scraping could convince him to use his wheelchair.

Personality changes ensued, like talking during church. Willie's children chuckled when they recalled their own punishment for failing to keep quiet at Mass—their dad would immediately remove them from the church and, if that didn't work, resort to spanking. Yet this Willie thought nothing of turning to Germaine as soon as a thought danced into his mind and discussing it with her, right in the middle of all the Hosannas. "Shhh. Behave yourself," she'd scold, more embarrassed than if it had been one of her small children breaking the rules.

Another personality change brought stubbornness and anger. Like the time he made his family repaint an entire room because they hadn't used the paint *he* had bought; they'd used Germaine's can of paint instead. It was the same color, just a different brand.

One morning, Germaine left the house, which irritated Willie so much that he hobbled to the door and locked it behind her. When she tried to get back in, she had to punch the doorbell repeatedly and pound on the door. No answer. Knowing full well the trouble Willie could get himself into, she started to panic. But finally, her now-102-year-old mother managed to move herself to the door with her walker and unlock it. Germaine glanced into the living room to see Willie plopped in a chair—only a few feet from the door she had been banging on—staring at the television set. It was, for Germaine, reminiscent of the time she took Willie to the support group and he made her wheel him to the restroom—whereupon he immediately locked himself in and wouldn't unlock it until forty-five minutes later when the meeting was over. Stubborn guy, that one.

And sneaky. Oh dear. While Germaine never objected to Willie's smoking, and even bought his cigarettes for him, she liked to keep track of him while he lit up, for fear he might burn the house down. But she later found out she wasn't his only supplier—he had also talked two neighbors into sneaking him cigarettes, as evidenced by all the packs and lighters, which she had not bought, sprinkled throughout his man cave in the garage.

Confusion soon set in. One day, Germaine walked into the bedroom and found her husband dumping jewelry into his hat. "And just what are you doing stuffing jewelry into your hat?" she asked Willie.

"Someone told me to do it," he said, shrugging. Fortunately, Willie took a nap later on, and Germaine seized that opportunity to hide her jewels from him. Later, she witnessed Willie searching through empty drawers with a flashlight, trying to figure out what had happened to his sparkling treasures.

It didn't take long for Germaine to realize that if she was going to survive her caregiving responsibilities, she would have to change the color of her lens. Willie had a mind of his own, and as his body continued to betray him, she knew that one of her top priorities would be to help him maintain his dignity.

So she learned to lighten up.

She reconciled herself to the fact that falls and awkward predicaments were an inescapable part of Willie's journey. She resolved not to compound his embarrassment by rebuking him for his foibles. She would be the resilient net beneath her husband.

Germaine was now serving as fulltime caregiver, not just for Willie, but for her mother, too. Ruby, always robust for her age, was developing serious health problems. She was tumbling often, for one. After a particularly violent fall, Germaine realized she was unable to care for her mother adequately. Ruby went to stay in a transitional care center, which was a huge loss for both Germaine and Willie.

A month later, Willie began his descent into dementia. Disturbing dreams and erratic behavior, compounded by blurry eyesight and double vision plagued him. Finally, a bout of pneumonia and two broken ribs from a fall out of bed sent him to the hospital. With that setback, he left home, never to return again. Willie ended up in the same care facility, and on the same floor, as Ruby. Germaine now had two people to visit at the center, but at the same time, she got her helpmate back. Ruby was able to shuffle over and visit Willie often, providing him familiarity in a strange place.

One day, Germaine walked in on the two of them playing together at the nurses' station. Willie had spread the contents of his favorite toy, a bucket of large, plastic nuts and bolts of various sizes, all over the counter. He reached over and grabbed Ruby's plastic pieces, scolding, "Give them to me. You don't know how to do it." Ruby responded with her typical good nature. When Germaine saw the two interacting, she knew she was only half of Willie's caregiver package. Ruby was—and had been all along—the other half.

Much to her chagrin, Germaine watched her formerly pleasant, amenable husband become combative, even abusive in his new surroundings. He didn't sleep, he wouldn't stay in bed, and he was able to escape any restraint the nurses could come up with, usually ending with his lying on the ground in a heap. The staff assigned him temporarily to a place near the nurses' station like a troublemaker in a classroom, and gave him a beanbag chair to sit on so his falls would be closer to the ground. He was supervised and strongly medicated until finally, the facility found a permanent solution: they padded the floor of an entire room and let him do whatever he wanted in there. Germaine breathed more easily after that—she had been terrified they'd assign him to a psychiatric hospital.

But there was no escaping the inevitable. When Willie was no longer able to urinate, when he had to have his kidneys drained, when he became irreparably disoriented, and when drooling was his main affect, Germaine knew what she had to do. She entreated the help of a dear and experienced friend from her support group to walk her through her options and the next step she needed to take for Willie: hospice.

Willie's first day in the hospice facility was nightmarish. He fought the staff all night long. But when Germaine arrived in the morning, he was clean and sleeping peacefully—for the first time in months. Just four days later, two weeks after their twenty-fifth wedding anniversary, Willie died. As he had requested, his brain was recovered for research at the Mayo Clinic.

Several months after Willie passed, Germaine wound up in the hospital again, this time with signs of a heart attack. A month of tests on every part of her body resulted in a diagnosis that would surprise few:

stress and depression. But it didn't sound right to Germaine. "I didn't feel sad," she says. "I never resented taking care of Willie. How could I have been depressed?" As she later learned, many of her fellow caregivers became ill after their loved ones passed on. The wisdom of her experience is universal: take care of yourself so you can take care of others.

Germaine mourned her loss deeply, but she still had her mother to take care of. Ruby, by now 104 years old, had been one of Willie's greatest fans, and she, too, felt great loss. Before Ruby's death more than a year later, Germaine was talking to her about heaven. "You'll be with all the people you loved again."

Ruby puckered her brow. "Yes, but will Willie be there?"

"Of course he will, Mother." With that, Ruby could rest in peace.

And Germaine herself lives out her own days in peace knowing she has her own personal caregivers looking out for her from their places in heaven: her mother and her perfect husband—John and Willie.

Barbara and Jerry

"Hard work doesn't have to mean being miserable."

Good morning, good morning, good morning,
it's time to rise and shine.
Good morning, good morning, good morning,
I hope you're feeling fine.
The sun is just above the hill, another day for
us to fill
With all the things we love to do!
Oh, can't you hear? It's calling you!

Barbara sauntered into the bedroom she shared with her husband, Jerry, just in time to start the second verse of their daily song. Her husband, immobile in the grips of multiple system atrophy, or MSA, lay with his mouth poised to join her. "Sing, even if all you can do is mouth the words," was part of his litany of self-help therapies.

Barbara beamed as she heaved his broad shoulders upright, pulled his stiffened legs one by one over the edge of the mattress, and propped him majestically onto his bed throne.

Jerry and Barbara still slept in the same bed—almost. Barbara had squished a twin bed right up next to Jerry's hospital bed, so they would be close enough to cuddle before falling asleep for the night. Often Barbara would doze off on his shoulder and he would have to awaken her because his arm had gone numb. Then she'd roll onto her own bed, close enough to his that she could adjust it as needed during the night to help him avoid bedsores.

With Jerry finally upright, Barbara turned to position his wheelchair.

She heard what sounded like a chuckle coming from Jerry. She turned around to see her athletic, hard-working, capable husband slowly,

41

slowly tipping backward onto the bed like a melting snowman. She giggled along with him.

Whoa. Wait a minute. Stop right there.

Are these people for real?

Jerry had MSA, for crying out loud, a devastating, debilitating neurological disease that was progressively robbing him of his power and identity. An illness that brought isolation, causing him to feel lonely day after day. A condition that heaped all manner of indignities upon him. And they were singing *I hope you're feeling fine?*

Barbara, a multitalented educator, systems organizer, and consultant in her own right, was now focused on meeting the needs of her husband every day, which was not always a pretty picture. *Another day for us to fill with all the things we love to do?* Oh, please.

The question bears repeating: all the beaming and giggling and cuddling—was that for real?

Well, yes and no. The journey to their acceptance of a new reality and their commitment to positivity was admittedly thorny at first. They had to learn in the trenches.

"I didn't accept my diagnosis well," acknowledged photographer, real estate developer, and minister Jerry. "I was in denial for a year. Then something switched inside, and I decided I would fight and overcome it. Both attitudes were normal, I suppose, but neither helped cure me."

It was a mild summery day in June when Jerry's first symptom appeared. He and Barbara were taking one of their frequent walks when an elderly couple approached them, holding hands and taking in the lush beauty. "That's us when we're old," said Barbara. Jerry smiled. But that day, Barbara sensed something different in her husband's gait. After more than thirty years walking side by side with him, she knew his pattern. *Something* was different.

Two months later, the couple were out walking again. Even though the day was hot, Jerry kept his hands in his pockets. "It helps me keep my balance," he responded to her confused query. *That's odd,* thought Barbara. But she brushed off her uneasy feeling.

As leaves abandoned their branches and westerly winds escorted winter over the mountains and into town, the couple took to walking the indoor track at the gym. One day, Barbara glanced briefly into the mirror as they passed and she noticed that Jerry's arm was stuck stiffly to his side. "Jerry, keep moving your arm," she said. "Do it purposefully. Keep thinking about it." He complied. But by the next lap, his arm was stiff again. *Well, everything else is normal,* she consoled herself. *He's the same old Jer.*

Then one final telltale sign came to Barbara's attention. "Jerry? Why have you been dictating everything to your secretary instead of typing it yourself?" she asked one day.

After a long silence, Jerry finally spoke. "I . . . can't write," he said.

Barbara's thoughts swarmed like pesky gnats as she tried to find a reasonable explanation for his terrifying symptoms. Well, he *has* been suffering from anxiety lately, she reasoned. After Hurricane Katrina, Jerry had been part of a team of city leaders that supervised the refurbishing of an old army barracks nearby, readying the empty rooms for over a thousand displaced storm victims. The tasks were myriad and challenging: coordinating cleaning crews, acquiring furniture, collecting clothing and personal hygiene items, preparing food, and organizing toy drives. He addressed everything from the spiritual needs of broken souls to the safety concerns of neighborhood schools. *That would be enough to assault the body with physical abnormalities,* Barbara thought.

But that wasn't it. Visits to neurologists resulted in three different diagnoses over a three-year span: first, dystonia, a disorder characterized by involuntary muscle contractions that cause slow, repetitive movements or abnormal postures; then two years later, Parkinson's disease; and finally, a year after that, multiple system atrophy.

As Jerry's caregiver for many years, Barbara was on a huge learning curve. She had this to say: "When a disease is progressive, we have time to research what we're in for, to absorb it, and to invent strategies and ways of coping simply out of necessity. The traditional wisdom—keep perspective, maintain balance, be prepared, use humor, remain flexible, foster positivity, live one day at a time—all of that sounds clichéd after a while. But the fact is that each of those wise nuggets is actually a skill that needs to be purposefully developed and steadily practiced. Jerry and I weren't automatically, by some mysterious force, filled with joy when we received his diagnosis. We've had to work at it—hard—every step of the way. Accepting that our life is different now was a journey in itself."

But hard work didn't have to mean being miserable, the two decided. Barbara and Jerry made a conscious decision to choose hopefulness as often as possible. That optimism would drive them to find ways to be happy even though their lives had taken a seemingly sinister turn. One of the best ways to beat negativity, they found, was to extend themselves to the people around them, and they made a commitment to make outreach a cornerstone of their lives.

Throughout Jerry's decline, he and Barbara grew in faith and wisdom. "When I made the decision that I had to fight this disease," said Jerry, "it initially led to hope, but eventually gave way to resolve. Now, my only hope is in God." It was during their battle with Jerry's disease that the couple finally learned optimism was their best recourse. Their only other choice was to drag each other down into the mire of self-pity, and they knew that was no way to live. Through trial and error, the couple learned some tips for what was helpful to them and what was not in their new, illness-defined life. In Jerry's words:

- I need respect. I'm an adult, so I would like you not to talk to me as if I were a child. I'm not mentally incapacitated just because I'm physically handicapped. You would be surprised at all the knowledge that's trapped inside my head.
- Allow me dignity in undignified situations, such as using the bathroom or getting dressed.
- Laugh with me to lighten the load.
- Grieve with me. The losses are real.
- My loneliness can be crushing at times. Getting out of the house and doing something productive helps the most, even if it's going to the doctor, running errands with Barbara, or being around people at the mall or at church.
- I would encourage my comrades in this fight not to deny themselves the simple pleasures of life. Laugh at least twice as much as you cry. Surround yourself with people and activities that were part of your life before the diagnosis. Fill your life with love and ice cream.

As Jerry's caregiver, Barbara knows the insight most dear to her husband's heart, the one that, once he grasped the profoundness of its meaning, brought him peace unlike any other strand of wisdom.

She quotes her husband: "Meditating on the scriptures brings me peace. I consider how good God is, that he is not angry with me, and that he still has a plan for my life exactly as it is."

Pat and Bob

"Life is good. It really is."

After caring for Bob in one capacity or the other during their entire forty years of marriage, Pat didn't think twice about her daily practices. After all, she'd married a man who'd been living with type 1 diabetes since he was eleven years old, so checking his blood sugar levels was about as routine as dusting the shelves. More recently, he'd had heart bypass surgery.

"But I have to admit," she says reluctantly, "This disease is whole different story."

Not that she was feeling sorry for herself. Not Pat. Not the woman who at age nineteen had to be strong for her mother after her brother was killed in a car accident. Not the young adult who, ten years later, lost her mother to colon cancer. Self-pity? Never. And not Bob either. Pfff—those two lived a life fuller than the Pillsbury Doughboy's gut. With no children to define their lifestyle, Bob and Pat let no dreams go unfed.

The couple met as neighbors, their apartments just across the hallway from each other. They would spend three years building a foundation of friendship before ever dating, but once they did, marriage followed without a blink. A fisheries biologist right out of college, Bob was driven by his type A personality, leadership skills, and outgoing nature to move into upper- management positions. Stints in the oil industry and, later, in environmental cleanup rounded out his career, and after devoting every ounce of energy he had to his job, he was able to retire at age forty-eight.

Through it all, Pat and Bob lived life to the fullest. Race cars were their thing. Years of tours, autocrosses, and high-speed driving events belied the Ken-doll persona of Pat's environmentalist husband. And she was right there next to him at most events. Memberships in a Porsche club and a vintage racing club surrounded them with a social group that fueled their passion.

In the midst of all their get-up-and-go, the changes in Bob came on gradually, slipping up on him like weeds in a carefully tended plot.

Zoning out.

Hands shaking.

Poor balance.

Stumbling.

Falling.

Increasingly low stamina, which caused him to quit his post-retirement travels with a professional race team.

Waning interest in all things formerly fun.

Visits to an endocrinologist came up with nothing. A series of tests by a neurologist—at Pat's insistence—proved more fruitful. Bob was likely suffering from Parkinson's disease, and physical therapy would best help him. But it didn't, because he wasn't.

Finally, seven years after the first signs of his deterioration appeared, Bob received a diagnosis that fit his symptoms: progressive supranuclear palsy. Once PSP crept into their lives and wrapped its crushing force around Bob, the couple watched their dream list dwindle. It wasn't long before every decision they made, every activity they planned, was at the whim of this neurological disease that wouldn't quit. As Pat explains, "Both our buckets had holes in them. We began to live moment by moment and rounded each corner as it came."

The couple were determined to live a quality life until their options were gone, but even that was difficult as time and time again a sickening fall would herald the arrival of new symptoms. One day, Pat and Bob drove to Sports Authority to buy walking sticks and sturdy shoes that they would use for the workout regimen they planned to start soon. They parked their car at the far end of the parking lot and headed for the store, wanting to get in a little exercise that very day. On the way back, Bob charged ahead of Pat. *Oh, it's wonderful seeing him run,* thought Pat optimistically. She picked up her speed to keep pace. But within seconds, she realized he wasn't running of his own volition.

Bob was out of control.

Suddenly, Pat had a slap-in-the-forehead moment. The memory of her husband explaining how he often had the sensation of racing downhill while walking exploded in her head, taunting her with its cruelty. *How could I have forgotten that?* She stood by helplessly as Bob headed for sure disaster.

Thud!

He plunged headfirst onto the pavement.

Gasps. Screams. A colorful blur of passersby rushed to help him. But Pat was at the head of the pack, cell phone in hand. Once again, the paramedics would earn the name she and Bob had dubbed them: BFFs, best friends forever. This time the cut over Bob's eye would cause optic nerve damage, and he would lose his sight on the left side.

Pat soon began to feel somewhat isolated in her caregiving role. No one was aware of the extent of Bob's deterioration, and no one could possibly fathom the complexity of her emotions. She was surprised to learn, therefore, that a support group, specifically for caregivers of people with PSP and another parkinsonism, multiple system atrophy, was awaiting her with open arms. It took only one meeting to realize she'd found a group who understood every nuance of her life with Bob, and she drew on their strength and compassion with fidelity. Bob, on the other hand, chose not to attend support group meetings with other people who had the disease. "There's no way I want to see where I end up," he asserted.

Pat learned from her fellow caregivers to put plastic urinals everywhere Bob went—the family room, the car, near his bed—so she wouldn't have to be constantly cleaning up the relics of his incontinence. It was also they who suggested installing grab bars between the bedroom and the bathroom so Bob could make his own way around. Among the other tips they gave her were rails around the toilet to prevent Bob from falling backward, and rugs at the bottom of the stairs to cushion his falls as he made his way up.

And it was out of their empathy that she accepted permission to let Bob fall. "Protecting Bob from himself was a challenge," says Pat. "And he got annoyed if I was there all the time, hovering. I learned from other caregivers that when you're not with them, you just wait for the thud. It's only a matter of time."

In an attempt to maintain her exercise regimen, Pat would walk with friends early in the morning while Bob still slept. Her plan worked beautifully—until the day she came home to find Bob asleep on the couch.

Earlier, he had walked himself into the living room and gone back to sleep. Figuring she had a few minutes before he woke up again, she decided to slip over to the coffee shop. When she returned not ten minutes later, she gasped. There was Bob, teetering at the top of the stairs, ready to topple backward. She caught him just in time. After that, she redefined her idea of leisure. Home-based activities such as knitting, baking cookies, and reading replaced the adventures she had grown accustomed to in her life with Bob.

Pat runs a hand through her gray, spiked hair.

"People think I should be bummed. Depressed. Miserable. But I'm honestly not. The fact is, this is our life now," she says.

"I've chosen to have a positive attitude and make the best of every day. I think each day starts out as a good day. Some go downhill very quickly but we recover and go on. I think it's important to look for and enjoy the good things in life. Perhaps the deer and the elk in the yard, some new plants coming up out of the snow, the frost and snow on the trees after a snow storm, a beautiful sunrise. All of these things feel good to me and serve as reminders on a regular basis that life is good. It really is."

Caring for Self

Deri and Beaver

"Any time spent rejuvenating oneself ultimately results in
more quality time to spend with the patient."

Deri looks toward the snow-capped mountains where scenes of her father busting his biking chops loom large in her childhood memories. "Beaver," she says, using the family's nickname for Lee, "was kind, patient, loving, and the best father anyone could ever ask for. He was a true hero in my eyes. I spent my childhood idolizing a man I thought could never fall. My dad was the most amazing man I know."

Deri shared her hero with her son, Zach, and her mother, Callae. As the daughter of both the patient and the caregiver, as well as the mother of a child who would lose his idol, Deri played a unique role in the family. Supporting Zach, Beaver, and Callae simultaneously, she was the caregiver who wore the three-cornered hat of psychologist, nurse, and proverbial "shoulder."

When the diagnosis of progressive supranuclear palsy, or PSP, entered the family's world, they knew absolutely nothing about it. They learned fast though. Devastated by the prognosis, each nevertheless held onto hope that the situation might take a different path—that Beaver wouldn't be a statistic, and he would live. It was the only way Deri could get through those first few months. The blessing of having such a rare, obscure disease was that the family couldn't possibly fathom what lay ahead for Beaver or for them. They simply lived their days one at a time and didn't look too far in the future.

One of Deri's first challenges was to figure out how to tell her five-year-old son that his hero was going to die. To Zach, Grandpa Beaver not only walked on water, he was the true Batman. What words would a five-year-old understand that wouldn't bring the crushing darkness she now knew into his innocent life?

Gradually, with Deri's support, Zach adjusted to a new normal.

His questions were profound for such a young child. Does PSP hurt? Is it contagious? Is Beaver sad? How will he die? What will Heaven be like? Will I see Grandpa Beaver there someday?

And his solutions were simple. "I'm going to be a scientist when I grow up," Zach asserted one day. "I'm going to discover a pill that Beaver can swallow and make the PSP go away."

A recurring conversation between Zach and Deri involved baseball. "If Beaver wasn't sick, would he play baseball with me in the yard?" asked Zach. Deri got down on her knees, looked her little boy in the eyes, and placed her hands on his thin shoulders. "You have no idea how much he would like to play with you, Zach. It would be a true gift."

Just as Deri tried to shield Zach, Beaver was protective of his daughter. He never once talked to her about his illness. In fact, he guarded her so fiercely that for a short period of time, she thought—just maybe— there was hope. Sadly, her nurse's training told her otherwise, and sure enough, weeks turned into months, one season bled into the next, and Beaver continued to decline. New physical changes appeared daily, yet Beaver repeated his mantra: "I'm doing just fine."

Indeed, Deri has countless happy memories of their days together, many infused with his contagious smile. Despite all the torment his body was going through, he still managed to pull his face into a grin and let out an occasional laugh, which consoled Deri like nothing else.

Still, her feelings bounced around like a bobber on a choppy lake. One day she'd feel buoyed by hope, the next, she'd sink into despair watching her dad struggle as he tried to stand, sit, speak, even swallow.

As Beaver's disease progressed and caregiving responsibilities increased, Deri could see the urgency of making sure she and her mother took care of themselves, too, by planning outings that brought them all respite. The family scheduled uplifting activities, both special and ordinary—picnics in the mountains, visits to the natural history museum, or just quiet time on the patio watching Zach play with the dogs. They would laugh as often as possible and feel as happy as they could for that moment.

The ease of staying active, however, was quickly coming to an end for Beaver. He was having more and more trouble with his balance, and his eyesight was all but gone. "He fought getting a walker with every bone in his body," says Deri. "And for him, a wheelchair was even worse. But we knew that in order to keep both himself and my mom safe—not only for the outings, but even to just get to the bathroom—it was time."

To mitigate the indignity of it all, and to make it fun for everyone, Deri and her mother joined Beaver in coming up with comical names for each of the assistive devices he acquired over time. He had a cane named Stick Dog, a walker dubbed Flash, and when the dreaded wheelchair made its appearance, it acquired the moniker Big Green. Biblet was Beaver's daily bib, but his Christmas bib bore special elegance: it resembled the front of a tuxedo. Ignoring the food that didn't make it to Beaver's mouth, the family instead raved about his high style.

Deri watched her father become more and more like a child over the four years of his illness. He needed help doing most everything. Although she helped with his care as often as she could, she didn't have to endure the intensity of the day-in, day-out responsibilities her mother did. Deri felt helpless as her dad's care took its toll on her mother, so from time to time, Deri's husband would come stay with Beaver while she got her mother out of the house. But each time, a short while into their leisure activity, Callae would start checking her watch, her worry overshadowing their fun.

"Caregivers," says Deri without hesitation, "are saints. Mom did everything she could every single day in order to keep Dad at home. She was both physically and mentally exhausted. She was a walking zombie." In the course of Beaver's decline, Callae lost four clothing sizes and didn't even realize it. But day after day, she trudged on, lovingly and loyally caring for her husband. She felt that no one else could care for him the way she did. Worried for her mom, Deri sought help.

"It was about this time that I reached out for a support group for my family and me. I personally needed someone to walk with me during these horrible years sure to come, and I thought it would be helpful to Mom, too," says Deri. Her phone call to the PSP/MSA support leader, Daniel, was the best step she could have taken during Beaver's illness. Daniel gently answered the million questions she had and welcomed her and Callae into their group, where they found a place of unconditional support, unfiltered answers, and, as Deri describes it, "the beginning of a love for each other that goes so deep I can't describe it adequately."

Deri and Callae faithfully attended group meetings twice a month for the next few years. The sessions allowed them to feel some modicum of peace in the heartbreaking situation they all shared. Sometimes Deri would bring Zach if he was out of school so he, too, could be with others who could comfort him. But Beaver himself never went to a support group meeting. "I believe it was too hard for him to see others living with the disease that was robbing them all of a future. I think he was scared to get a glimpse of those patients further along than himself. He just said it wasn't his cup of tea, and we left it at that," says Deri.

Following the path of many of her new caregiver friends, and with Deri's encouragement and support, Callae finally agreed to enlist the help of a palliative care team. Deri's praise is effusive. "They came into my parents' home, helped Mom, gave her a break, and took amazing care of Dad," she says. "Just like our support group, the team became like family."

Deri's best advice for caregivers is to take care of themselves. "The PSP journey is a long one," she says with urgency. "Any time spent rejuvenating oneself ultimately results in more quality time to spend with the patient." Deri had watched too many caregivers succumb to both physical and emotional ailments, during or after their exhausting years attending to the needs of people with debilitating degenerative diseases, and she didn't want her mother to be a statistic.

When it became clear that Beaver's life was coming to an end, and the hospice team had set up a hospital bed in the living room so Beaver could feel a part of everyday life, Deri's anxiety began to increase. Her love for her father filled her every cell, and even when he could no longer speak, the bond was still palpable; their love for each other needed no words. But she was plagued with conflict, one she couldn't share with her dad: her father-in-law, who lived several states away, was also deathly ill, and it appeared his end was near. Her greatest fear was that her father-in-law was going to go first, taking Deri away from Beaver.

That was exactly what ended up happening. Before she flew to her father-in-law's funeral, she wrote her dad a letter and left it with Callae. What Beaver saw before he left this life were two pages filled with loving words from his daughter. He learned that in Deri's eyes, he had been the perfect father. He saw how heartbroken she was that this illness had devoured him like the beast it was. He read that Deri would miss him from the very depths of her being, that she would never let Zach forget him, and that Callae would be okay—she would see to that.

But knowing her dad had seen her letter was no consolation when she got word from far away that Beaver was actively dying. Unable to disguise the pain in her heart, she boarded the plane for her flight back home, trying to make the aircraft fly faster by simply wishing it to do so. Torn between her horrific sadness and her gratefulness that her dad's four-year ordeal of suffering was almost over, she headed back to her hero.

She got home just in time. The warm, gentle Indian summer outdoors mirrored the peace that filled the living room, beckoning Deri inside. Beaver's closest loved ones had gathered. But when he took his final breath, it was Deri who was right by his side, holding his hand. Beaver had waited for his only daughter, the one he always called his favorite.

The blur that followed Beaver's death still plays through Deri's mind in slices of images, like a movie trailer:

Zach releasing a host of monarch butterflies at the celebration of his grandfather's life.

The sights and smells of her father in her parents' home that lingered after his passing.

The small doses of peace that managed to sneak in and find Deri, though not often enough.

Sessions at Footprints, the grief-counseling program for children offered by hospice.

Zach's frequent, almost mystical conversations with his grandpa, and his matter-of-fact announcements that "Beaver is here."

And the Miracle Bears, sewn by a family in Oklahoma, whose mission it was to offer solace to grieving families by crafting teddy bears out of the deceased's clothing.

One day, Deri, Zach, and Callae were rummaging through Beaver's clothes trying to find something that would make a good bear, one that would embody the man they loved. Although Deri and her mother wanted to use some nice shirts that flooded them with memories of Beaver in a healthier time, Zach would have none of it. That wasn't how he remembered his hero. Instead, he chose clothing that typified the only grandfather he knew: his Miracle Bear would wear a white T-shirt, sweatpants, and a hoodie.

Just like Beaver.

JoAnn and Fred

"Travel seemed like the best way to keep us both interested in life."

In the face of most any problem, JoAnn took care of herself by creating fun. Take the valley in her life, for example, when sadness after sadness descended upon her like smog on a stifling day: first her dad died, then she had a cancer scare and subsequent lumpectomy, then her husband, Fred, grew discontent with his job, and the couple had to move from the home they loved. In the convergence of so much trial all at once, JoAnn became depressed. So what did she do? She spearheaded an invasion of alligators throughout downtown.

"The college students I knew used to say, 'When you're up to your ass in alligators, it's hard to remember the mission was to drain the swamp.' So I decided to have a little fun with those beasts," says JoAnn. She and her team of fellow mischief-makers used donated fabric and paint to fashion their life-sized alligators, and weeks later, the toothy heads peeked out of storm drains, slithered over bridges, and stopped frenzied workers in their tracks as they scurried across busy downtown streets. Despite three days of television coverage, including an interview with JoAnn—her face hidden at her request—the self-effacing woman managed to stay in the background. "I just wanted some fun," she says.

JoAnn brought that same sense of fun into caregiving. It helped that Fred's deterioration came in gradual steps. It helped that they were still able to maintain their emotional connection. It helped that they could laugh and tease and even flirt occasionally.

After all, the relationship almost never happened.

JoAnn and Fred worked for the same company and spoke with each other on occasion. But it wasn't until a chance meeting in the supermarket that Fred stepped out of his business demeanor and approached JoAnn on a personal level. The handsome, well-dressed Mensa genius, known for his compassion and integrity, who would one day be flying around the world in corporate jets, heading up uranium and copper mines, and eventually founding a solid, successful investment firm with millions of dollars in assets, had a question for his spunky, diminutive coworker: "How do you cook broccoli?" The culinary discussion and chitchat that followed revealed that they lived just a block from each other, which led to their first date, a trip to the zoo to see an art show.

But her bubble burst that day. Fred's constant complaining about work, his walking away when he saw her moved to tears by a poetic reading, and his incredibly unromantic move of buying—for himself—a painting she had said she herself wanted led her to mutter under her breath, "This is nobody I want to be with."

Yet less than a year later, JoAnn and Fred were married. "It was the harmonica," she says. "He invites me over to sunbathe on his roof and he hauls out a harmonica, of all things. That analytical little jerk cares enough to play the harmonica. That did it for me."

But what truly sealed the deal for JoAnn was what she calls their "biblical experience." It was also the moment when it looked like Fred was going to be the caregiver of the two: she had a health condition she hadn't mentioned to him. She woke up one morning in Fred's apartment to see that a bird had flown through an open window. Perched on the bureau, the feathered visitor filled the room with its angelic warble, awakening Fred from his slumber. As JoAnn tells it, "It was a magical moment, almost biblical. And I realized that after you're biblical with someone, you have to be completely honest. I told Fred I was going to have surgery for suspected cancer."

What did Fred do? He proposed to JoAnn. "If it's bad cancer, we'll just travel till you die," he promised. The couple married at a large downtown church with just her father, the pastor, and the cleaning lady present.

But Fred didn't have to be the caregiver after all. JoAnn came through her surgery with a good bill of health, and the couple spent the next twenty-eight years twirling in a dance of travel, entrepreneurship, friendships, and family bonding. They were soul mates in every way.

No, Fred never had to be a caretaker for his wife. Quite the opposite.

His voice was the first thing to go.

Driven in every area of his life—graduating college in two years at age eighteen, excelling at tennis, skiing, hiking, fishing, and just about anything he attempted—Fred watched helplessly as his voice weakened. In a short period of time it went from a powerful tool in his occasional role as confident pontificator—dominating the conversation after a couple of drinks—to no sound at all. His physician finally sent him to a speech therapist. It didn't help. The deterioration was underway.

A year later, Fred made the hardest decision of his life: he stopped working. His difficulty concentrating, the "brain blips" he suffered that impeded his ability to make connections, and his uncharacteristic lack of ambition were mystifying, but undeniable. Even harder than the physical limitations was Fred's emotional state. A sponge for knowledge and a magnet for possibilities, Fred had dedicated his life to creating projects and bringing them to fruition with aplomb. Now, no ambition. Worse, no doctor seemed to know what was happening to him.

The next year, JoAnn was by his side as they listened to the perplexed neurologist. "You're not falling into any of the typical categories," he said as he closed Fred's file. "I'm going to refer you to the Mayo Clinic." The solemn tone in his voice hit JoAnn in the gut; this was even more serious than she'd feared. The neurologists at the Mayo Clinic found Fred's condition equally challenging. Their closest assessment was olivopontocerebellar atrophy, the degeneration of neurons in specific areas of the brain—the cerebellum, pons, and inferior olive.

Back home again, the news didn't get any better. Fred's neurologist prescribed Sinemet, to no effect. And the speech therapist announced that she couldn't help Fred anymore. She suggested the couple use a speech machine so Fred could type what he wanted to say and let the machine do the talking. But eventual loss of finger dexterity put an end to even this small luxury.

Finally, four years after Fred's first disturbing symptoms, the medical search ended. Fred received an official diagnosis: progressive supranuclear palsy. At last, JoAnn knew what she was dealing with. She was now a caregiver for her terminally ill husband who would deteriorate, sometimes quickly, sometimes slowly, sometimes all at once. There was no cure, no return to their former life.

"We'll just travel till you die," Fred had pledged to JoAnn thirty-

JUST LISTEN FOR THE THUD

two years before. Now it was JoAnn's turn. Indeed, travel seemed like the best way to keep both of them interested in life. It was also a healthy escape for her. So the same year Fred's diagnosis tried to bury the couple's joyful, productive life in its volcanic ash, JoAnn and Fred planned a trip to China.

Thud. Shortly before their departure, Fred fell and bruised his ribs. But the couple was undeterred. A bottle of pain pills followed them to Asia—as did Fred's tendency to tip backward. JoAnn and Fred quickly learned to see the light side of their plight, however. While Fred immersed himself completely into the experience of China, JoAnn—and other tourists in the group—quickly became skilled at leaping to Fred's rescue whenever he started to tip over.

People were kind when they saw JoAnn needed assistance, and she was learning that keeping herself well meant accepting all the help she could get. One day, on the return flight from China, Fred got up to use the bathroom. Suddenly he tumbled to the floor, creating a brouhaha that rivaled a pulsating emergency room. Flight attendants rushed to pull Fred up off the floor, move passengers, clear a row, and lay him across the seats.

"What happened here?"

JoAnn turned to see a tall, lean gentleman peering over the row where Fred lay. "I'm Dr. Dave," the man said. She soon learned that the physician worked in Wichita, Kansas, where JoAnn often visited her brother. That surprise brought an instant bond—and a feeling of security. Her sigh of relief was audible when Dr. Dave offered to keep an eye on Fred for the rest of the flight.

By the next year, Fred was confined to a wheelchair. His days were now filled with light exercises, acupuncture and massage, and plenty of rest. JoAnn transformed the main level of their house into a hospital. She replaced the laundry appliances with a walk-in bathtub, bought a high-quality lift chair, and surrounded him with magazines, newspapers, and a television set with a remote control. A skilled cook, JoAnn changed her entrees from attractive displays of beef bourguignon and coq au vin to blended food that resembled Dickensian gruel just so Fred could swallow without choking. The throbbing strobes of the ambulance outside their home became a common sight as paramedics raced in day and night to lift Fred after his falls.

JoAnn's life was drastically different now, but she embraced caregiving with an open heart. "You would never do this if you didn't truly love the person," she told friends.

Despite all the drastic changes, JoAnn did everything she could to make Fred's life meaningful and stimulating. Travel had always been one of his favorite activities, and, despite all the extra preparations it now took, travel was respite for her, too. A train trip across several states, a road trip to visit their nearly one-hundred-year-old friend, a trip out of the country. Short trips, long trips—they did it all.

One of their journeys was nearly catastrophic. JoAnn packed the vehicle, including all of Fred's necessary paraphernalia, and pointed the car in the direction of her brother's out-of-state home. Always aware of allowing Fred to be as independent as possible, she thought nothing of it when Fred was upstairs in her brother's guest room changing his clothes. Suddenly, *thud!* JoAnn raced up the steps to find her husband crumpled on the floor, having fallen forward against the doorframe of the closet. Frantic, she hurried to pick him up, dress him, grab a bag of ice for his aching neck, and get him into the car for the trip to the urgent care center.

"What happened here?" the tall, lean doctor asked. At the sound of the familiar voice, JoAnn was again flooded with relief. There to examine her husband's x-rays was Dr. Dave. "We met on the plane," she reminded him, hardly fazed by the unlikely coincidence.

"Oh, I *thought* I had treated Fred before," he said. "The plane ride from China. That was it."

And then he looked at the images. "My God," said Dr. Dave. "Let's get him in an ambulance stat. He has a broken neck." He looked JoAnn in the eye. "He could have died from this injury." Emergency personnel were waiting for Fred at the hospital to stabilize then treat him. Fortunately, his trip home was compliments of his travel insurance, which included a patient advocate to accompany him right to his front door.

A year later, JoAnn and Fred were back in the travel saddle again. This time it was a Mediterranean cruise. Twelve ports of call in twelve days, and Fred and JoAnn got off at each and every one. She had to feed Fred, and she did so unselfconsciously, even facilitating his intake of beer in Florence—his sippy cup and straw simply part of their traveling supplies. Strangers helped them without hesitation, pushing his wheelchair, carrying it up and down stairs, picking him up when he fell. Fred was ecstatic under the nurturing care of the warm Mediterranean sun, the sight and smell of the cerulean sea filling him with a sense of wellbeing. JoAnn felt nurtured, too.

The last year of Fred's life—six years after his first symptom appeared and two years after his diagnosis—saw him sixty pounds lighter, limited to holding up one or two fingers to communicate, and oscillating between frustration and depression. Countless Heimlich maneuvers saved him from choking to death. Falls were frequent, and JoAnn got to know her neighbors intimately as she knocked on their doors day and night to ask for help hefting her husband off the floor.

Gradually, Fred prepared to let go. By then, hospice staff had been providing services to Fred twice a week. He and JoAnn brought a new dog into their home so JoAnn would have company and comfort after Fred was gone. "What should we name our pet?" she asked. With the help of the letters on a Ouija board, Fred named the dog. His atrophied hands pushed the lightweight planchette across the board, letter by letter, spelling out his suggestion: Ginger.

And then something remarkable happened. Three days before his death, Fred got his voice back. He was especially intent on planning his Celebration of Life. He spoke in detail about what he wanted: the minister, the venue, the guests, the band, his favorite foods. He talked about how proud he was of his children, Steve, Sheryl, and Karla. He spoke of the people he loved. It was a rush of words that gushed from his mouth like a geyser. His thoughts flowed for an hour—no more, no less—then retreated to the confines of his recalcitrant brain once again.

Fred's children, knowing the end was near, came to be with their father. On his last day, they glued themselves to the chairs next to the hospital bed in the living room, where they squabbled good-naturedly over what song their father would want to hear. Finally, they turned on the music. Fred, his eyes glazed, slowly lifted his hand to give a fist pump. All was right in his world.

In the ensuing quiet and calm, Fred took his last breath.

With serenity, JoAnn reflects on her husband's final moment. "I've witnessed quite a number of people die," she says. "Fred's was as good a death as I've been through."

Callae and Lee

"People assumed I needed to get away. That's not what I wanted at all."

Callae's aircraft technician and safety inspector husband had bragged he would still be working when he was a hundred years old. But now, hobbling around on the cane he needed just to perform his basic job duties, he was ready to leave it all behind. Something was wrong with his body. Perhaps being in his relaxing home and having time to take walks at his whim would help him heal. Lee made the decision to retire, and a short while later, Callae followed.

The couple would spend the next two years trying to figure out what was happening to Lee. His symptoms were baffling, even scary at times.

Just to reassure themselves, Callae and Lee paid a visit to their internist, who suggested Lee might have "foot drop," a general term for difficulty lifting the front part of the foot. While the indicators looked suspiciously like progressive supranuclear palsy, or PSP, the internist was cautious and didn't want to alarm anyone by speculating on that diagnosis. So he kept it to himself and sent Lee home with some exercises to do.

When Lee's foot drop didn't improve, his internist referred him to a movement disorder specialist at the university's Health Sciences Center, who immediately diagnosed Lee with PSP. She then invited Lee's entire family, as well as Callae's, to take part in a nationwide research study attempting to find a cause for PSP and other degenerative neurological diseases. Her study focused on environmental factors such as long-term exposure to toxins like farm pesticides and aircraft fumes—exactly Lee's life up until then. They felt a flicker of hope. But although they participated, the family never heard the results of the study, and they were left to ponder the mystery of Lee's deteriorating condition.

Once Lee knew how sick he was, he did everything he could to be self-reliant. His trip to the barber was one such example. While Callae usually drove him, he got up the gumption one day to insist on driving himself. It wasn't far, nor did he need to get on any busy streets, he argued. Callae's knuckles went white as she reluctantly assented, then she stood by the window until he returned. When he walked in the door, he greeted her with a heart-stopping observation: "Boy, it's kind of hard when there are other cars on the street."

That was the last time Callae allowed herself to be filled with such terror. "You have to think about other people, Beaver," she said, using her term of endearment for him. "You don't want to be responsible for killing someone." After that, Lee allowed his wife to drive him for haircuts—but he wouldn't let her go in with him.

"He needed his independence," says Callae. "You can't just take all those things away at once."

Lee was also bent on keeping up his duties around the house. He was sure it would be fine to mow the lawn, for example; he had a John Deere riding mower, for heaven's sake. What could possibly go wrong? But Callae was uneasy. So she got two small, electric push mowers, one for each of them, and together they cut the grass.

Until the time Lee took a tumble.

Callae shrieked when she saw her husband splayed on the lawn, his glasses broken, the lawnmower on top of him with its blades spinning dangerously close to his body. *No more!* she screamed inside, and immediately hired someone to mow their lawn from that day on.

The saddest moment for Callae came the day they went to their daughter's home for dinner. Throughout the evening, Lee kept disappearing into the bathroom. Callae was confused, but this was no time to talk about it. On their drive home, though, Lee explained sadly, "I was feeling like I had to go the whole time, but it just wouldn't come."

As soon as they walked in the door, Lee headed straight for the bathroom. Callae followed a few minutes later and when she entered the room, she was shocked. There stood her husband, his urine all over the floor. She quickly cleaned it, but when she looked up, her heart shattered. Tears were streaming down Lee's cheeks as he uttered the words, "I think I'm losing control of my bladder. I'm just a pain in the ass to everyone."

"This disease robs them of all that's important to them," says Callae. "Lee was always able to take care of everything, and now he was powerless over his own body. Our hearts were simply broken. We held each other and both of us cried and cried."

Callae knew that if she wanted to take care of Lee, she would need to take care of herself. One thing she did faithfully was attend a support group for caregivers. "I'm not exaggerating when I say it was my lifeline," she says. The twice-monthly meetings, one of which was a social luncheon, gave her the feeling she wasn't alone. She was surrounded by people who understood and who cared, and by people who could help her lighten up. "Laughter is so important," she says. "I had to find things that would give Lee levity or we were both going to crash."

Callae reflects on her four years as Lee's caregiver. "People kept telling me I needed to bring in help so I could get away several times a week. I realize some people need that, but I didn't want that at all. I wanted to be with Lee. Who wouldn't want to spend time with such a kind, thoughtful man? We said 'I love you' more in the last year than in the previous ten. That's what gave me comfort."

She's emphatic when she says, "You can never judge what people should be doing for themselves. It's different for everyone."

Nevertheless, as time went on and Lee was falling more often, his internist talked to the couple about enlisting the help of a palliative care team. "This isn't the 'you-have-to-die-in-six-months' hospice situation," he assured them. He turned toward Lee. "This is a group of professionals, Lee, who will give you periodic checkups so you don't have to come see me all the time."

He could see Lee wasn't convinced. "And it will help Callae out," he added. That was all Lee needed to hear. If he couldn't take care of things himself, he wanted to make sure Callae had the support she needed. He looked at his wife with his big blue eyes, then at the doctor, then cemented the deal. "Well, if she needs help, that's okay," he said.

There were many more thuds as time went on, and as Callae tried to lift Lee's dead weight with less and less success, the paramedics grew into friends. Callae became a pro at tapping her husband's back to loosen phlegm and using the suctioning machine to clear him out. His swallowing difficulties prevented him from eating, and even from drinking at times.

The palliative team sent him heavier liquids like Ensure and thickened water. But Lee had an opinion about that. "Thickened water," he made it known, "is wrong. It's just wrong."

By the time Lee lost his battle, he was under the care of traditional hospice professionals and spending his days and nights in a hospital bed in the family room. Callae slept right beside him on the sofa for several months. Lee made it known when he was ready to give up the fight: he stopped eating, wouldn't take water, and started sleeping all day.

It was clear he was slipping away.

Callae was anxious because their only child, Deri, was out of town attending the funeral of her father-in-law, and she knew their daughter would be devastated if her dad died while she was gone. Still, the house began to fill with supportive people. Friends from out of state had come in, as had JoAnn, a dear friend from the caregivers' support group, whose own husband had lost the battle with PSP earlier. Once JoAnn arrived at the house, the crew was in place and ready for action like an orchestrated bucket brigade. Everyone knew what to do, and if they didn't, they learned fast.

Callae urged Deri to catch an earlier flight, then arranged to have Deri's best friend pick her up at the airport and bring her home to Lee. Callae kept vigil over her husband, sitting next to him on the bed, listening to his irregular breathing. And then a startling thought reverberated through her mind: *Oh my gosh. Maybe it's really going to happen. Maybe Lee is really going to die.* She was stunned at the thought and equally shocked that this moment was the first time she'd seriously entertained the idea that Lee might permanently leave her. As physically exhausted as she was from caregiving, she wasn't ready to let him go.

At bedtime, JoAnn urged Callae to get some sleep. JoAnn then sat all night at Lee's side, following hospice's protocol to a T, administering antianxiety medication and morphine, just as she had for her own husband. Every so often she implored Lee to hang on a little longer. "Deri is on her way, Beaver. She's almost here. Hang on."

At dawn, Callae resumed her post at her husband's side, the ticking of the clock punctuating the silence. Lee's time was drawing closer. She glanced nervously at the clock.

Morning had barely glided into afternoon when suddenly

the door burst open. "I'm here, Daddy! I'm here." Deri flew to her father's side.

Together, mother and daughter kept watch over the man who had so blessed their lives.

Breathing, slow breathing. Stop.

Breathing, slow, slow.

Stop.

And then, as peacefully as a sailplane aloft, Lee left his earthly mission behind.

Helenn and Joe

"Doing for someone else was far healthier than closing myself off from meeting people."

"You did what?" chided Helenn's frustrated father, waving the report card at his University of Illinois daughter. "I sent you to college to earn a sensible degree, Helenn, one that would get you a dependable job. What made you think you could switch your major without letting me know?"

"Well, I knew you would say no." Helenn straightened her plaid, pleated skirt. How could she explain her need to follow her dreams? Every woman she knew—if she went to college at all—was headed for a career in nursing, teaching, or scribbling shorthand. But a degree in radio and television would be Helenn's ticket out of the ordinary. She was certain she'd be successful in her chosen career. After all, TV, though still in its infant stages, was sure to follow the path of radio in its popularity and viability, perhaps even surpass it.

"Hear my words," said her father, forcing his knowledgeable persona. "This television thing is a passing fancy."

But the "television thing" swept Helenn right into a life beyond anything she could have imagined. A career woman when women didn't talk that way, Helenn took a job as a writer at WTVO in Rockford, Illinois, after graduation.

And that's when she met Joe.

The gregarious Notre Dame graduate of the Journalism School of Radio and Television was known not only for his success in sales, but for his sense of humor. Helenn was drawn to both those qualities. The only problem was, she didn't get his jokes. She got around this by telling her cohorts, "Now, when Joe comes in and tells a joke, laugh. Loudly." That's how she would know his repartee was complete, and she could join in the laughter.

Joe and Helenn fell in love, but their wedding vows would have to wait until after her two-year stint in Europe, where she was writing for the newspaper *Stars and Stripes*. Upon her return to the United States, she and Joe got married while they were both working for the NBC affiliate in Rockford, WRVO. A move to Seattle followed, then another to Denver—while they both climbed the ladder of that "passing fancy" like Cirque du Soleil acrobats.

By then, they had a son who craved their attention. Feeling moved to quit her job, but cringing at the image of her father tapping on her shoulder and saying, "See? It's not working out, is it?" Helenn chose a more family-friendly profession. She became a teacher, advocating for gifted and talented children.

Joe continued his ascent in the world of television, rising from successful salesman to successful local sales manager to successful national sales manager to successful general manager and president of TV stations in both Denver and Minneapolis. With his job came travel all over the world for the couple, as well as a robust social life. Adventures Helenn never knew as a child were suddenly hers, including helicopter rides from her home in suburban Minneapolis to Winter Carnival activities in St. Paul—just to avoid rush hour traffic.

Clearly, Joe was at the top of his field, having found a profession that enabled him to leave his mark. After he retired, he looked forward to an exciting and meaningful journey into a hard-earned life of leisure.

And then it all started to collapse.

He was falling regularly. At first he kept it to himself, but soon Helenn started to notice. The balance problems. The lack of spontaneity. Diminished congeniality. Yet nothing irregular showed up on the MRI his first neurologist ordered; she felt that Joe's problems were probably just due to normal aging. Symptoms continued to develop, however.

On the day Joe wandered across the golf course looking for the ball he missed, his golf partner, who was a heart specialist, approached Helenn. "I'm not a neurologist," he said, "but I know this is *not* normal aging." Helenn knew she would need to consult with experts trained in all types of neurological problems.

It was at the Mayo Clinic that Joe received a firm diagnosis:

progressive supranuclear palsy, PSP. Helenn was stunned. She'd never heard of this disease, never known anyone who'd suffered from it, and was having difficulty grasping what the progression would really look like. Over the course of the next five years, she found out: Joe lost all mobility, including the ability to speak, swallow, walk, and turn over.

As Joe's health presented more and more challenges, Helenn's role shifted from being his travel, social, and career partner to fulltime caregiver.

But Helenn was no victim. That had never been her style. Not the young coed, barely out of childhood, who took it on herself to stand in her truth and change her major all those years ago. Not the career woman who rose to success on her own terms. She had grit then, and she had it now.

Certainly, she felt discouragement at times, particularly when she could see the frustration in her brilliant husband, a member of Mensa, as he tried to negotiate his days with all his intelligence, ideas, and problem-solving skills locked inside his brain, unable to find expression. But she developed the philosophy that the only way to live in the uncertainty of life was to take advantage of every moment. She expressed gratitude for the life she and Joe had shared for so many years, and savored all their memories. She was thankful he had left so much of the business duties to her so she could continue them after his death. She treasured her son and granddaughter, who lived nearby. She had much to be grateful for.

Helenn didn't ignore her grief in the face of Joe's decline, but she allowed her sense of levity to carry her. She made the decision to see humor where she could, especially when it popped its head up in the midst of chaos, like a clown in a jack-in-the-box. It truly was a decision, as it wasn't always easy. Joe, too, kept his spirits raised as best he could. Throughout his illness, he never showed anger or belligerence, never grumbled or even complained. Yet he was fully aware of the nature of his journey.

One day, his close friend asked, "Joe, you've never complained. Why?"

Joe's answer was immediate. "The only thing I can say is that we all have to leave this life, and *something* is going to make that happen. My something is PSP. I've had one hell of a ride on earth. I have no regrets. It's just my time."

Helenn was Joe's primary caregiver until he expelled his last breath—at home and very much unexpectedly. She had no idea he was so close to death that day. With transfers from the hospital to a nursing home and back home again, no staff got to know him well enough to predict the end was near. But he was at home and she was with him, and that had been her greatest wish.

Even the aftermath of Joe's death took Helenn by surprise. She had prepared herself as well as a person could, but what she wasn't prepared for was the deep depression that buried her like a murky mudslide. Despite invitations to some of the familiar fundraisers and social gatherings she and Joe had attended together for years, those couples' events became extremely difficult for her and she simply could not garner the wherewithal to attend. Consequently, her formerly active life shriveled up, a once-vibrant bouquet now a dried petal.

Helenn will not underplay the grip depression had on her, but she ultimately reached a point where she knew she had to take care of herself. She had to get out of the house and make a contribution.

"I realized with time that giving myself in service to others was far healthier than closing myself off from meeting people," she says. Remembering vividly the isolation she felt when Joe was first diagnosed with a disease so few had ever heard of, and recalling the sense of relief when she found a support group full of people who understood what she was going through as his caregiver, Helenn knew what her next step would be.

"I wanted to give back in some way," she says, "so I now facilitate the PSP and MSA support group. It's a place where I can offer what I know best: compassion, camaraderie, and shared experience."

Helenn glances at the pictures of Joe, a gallery of all the stages of his memorable life lined up on shelves.

"It keeps me from having a pity party," she muses.

And with that, her smile returns.

Receiving Help

Carolyn and Dave

"They say God doesn't give us more than we can handle. Well, he gave me a turkey platter, put a cow on it, and thought I could carry it all!"

I t was a cloudy spring Saturday, and Carolyn was enjoying a welcome break from her busy schedule. In addition to her fulltime job, she was immersed in massage school. But Saturdays were catch-up time, and she appreciated that her husband, Dave, was out and about, giving her several hours of much-needed quiet time.

Suddenly, the shrill blare of the telephone broke her reverie. Its very bossiness irritated her. *Maybe I just won't answer it,* she thought. But her better judgment prevailed.

"Oh my gosh!" Carolyn's words echoed through an empty house. "I'll be right there." Her heart pounded as she raced to find her keys.

Dave had been in an accident.

When she got to the hospital, she found Dave lying in his bed, looking dazed.

He was frightened and confused. "I can't figure out how it happened," he said. "I was driving, getting ready to turn, then suddenly the car flipped over on its side." But it got worse. Because his speech was slurred, his demeanor awkward, the police concluded he had been driving under the influence.

The incident hit Carolyn smack in the face. She had noticed changes in Dave's speech and gait, but they were so gradual and so slight that she hadn't given them much thought. Now those peculiarities had garnered an undeserved presumption from law enforcement.

Carolyn brought Dave home, then spent the rest of the afternoon reviewing the past year in her mind.

There was the time he'd come home early from skiing, discouraged that his skills weren't up to par. "I just wasn't very coordinated today," he'd said. Carolyn had assured him that it was probably due to icy conditions, and encouraged him to try again the next day.

And then there was the time he'd asked Carolyn to show him how to use QuickBooks. She was baffled at his difficulty understanding the software, this man who could usually figure out most anything. *He must have a lot on his mind,* she'd thought. *He's distracted, that's all.*

She remembered, too, her sister's observation that, after not having seen Dave for a year, his affect was noticeably different. The normally gregarious Dave seemed subdued, distant. Carolyn herself hadn't noticed, but she tucked her sister's comment into the back of her mind.

And that tumble he'd taken. Startled by the thud, she ran outside to find that Dave had fallen off the garage steps. But falling was understandable when it was icy and cold outside, wasn't it?

For every aberration, there had always been a reasonable explanation.

Even his recent career change was beginning to take on new meaning in Carolyn's mind. At the time, she'd thought nothing of her husband's announcement that he was leaving politics once and for all to open a pet care business. The force behind the election of countless political figures, Dave had been growing increasingly disillusioned with the dog-eat-dog world he'd been a part of for thirty years. As a boy, he'd worked as a sheepherder, so it seemed logical to Carolyn that his post-retirement career would involve animals. His time, apparently, had arrived.

What Carolyn had no way of knowing was that these seemingly benign lifestyle and personality changes were the beginning of a life she could never have imagined.

And yet, even as mysterious symptoms were popping up like prairie dogs in a dusty field, Dave was moving forward with his second career. He obtained certification from the Animal Behavior College as a canine obedience trainer and became a certified volunteer instructor for pet first aid with the American Red Cross. For several years, he volunteered in an animal center's Psychology, Health, and Training program, working with dominant animals and dogs that had been in the shelter for long periods. And he poured himself into building his professional pet services business.

Then, on an overcast January afternoon, the couple found

themselves in the office of a neurologist who had conducted extensive tests on Dave. Though anxious, Carolyn was eager to get some kind of diagnosis. Not knowing was more stressful than knowing, no matter what she was going to hear. The good news, the doctor reported, was that the tests had eliminated the presence of a tumor or the possibility of a stroke. She suspected parkinsonism, which, she explained, was any condition that caused a combination of the movement abnormalities seen in Parkinson's disease, such as tremor, slow movement, impaired speech, or muscle stiffness. While not a diagnosis they cherished, they were relieved to know that Dave's symptoms were real; they hadn't imagined them.

The neurologist referred the couple to a movement disorder specialist for further exploration. Three hours with the second physician proved to be a watershed event for Dave and Carolyn. His conclusion: Dave had progressive supranuclear palsy. They had no idea what that meant. They simply put one foot in front of the other and moved forward with direction from their doctor. Physical therapy, increased medication, and treatments by a neurophysiologist gave them hope as Dave began to sleep better, longer, and more quietly.

Despite the distressing news, neither Carolyn nor Dave was willing to succumb to the role of victim. Both had full lives that refused to give power to this interruption.

Carolyn was glad Dave was so motivated and self-reliant because she soon fell into another challenging situation. Her mother, who lived out of state, had just received a diagnosis of pancreatic cancer, and Carolyn began traveling twice a month to see her. After working all week at her airline job, she would take a standby flight to the nearest large airport, rent a car, drive 105 miles to her mother's house, stay the weekend, and then retrace her journey. Then, yet another responsibility cropped up: not one, but both of her aunts fell seriously ill. Carolyn had no choice but to hand over her mother's care to her sisters while she took care of the two aunts. Still bound to her work schedule back home, she continued the two-hour flights back and forth on weekends to tend to them.

While all this was going on, Dave took a back seat to the out-of-town relatives. Although her husband was still self-sufficient, Carolyn felt guilty that she couldn't give him her full attention.

One day, she poured her heart out to her sisters. "They say God doesn't give us more than we can handle. Well, he gave me a turkey platter, put a cow on it, and thought I could carry it all! I think I'm finally getting the platter organized and making room for the cow, so I know I'll be fine." Realizing how her sisters had been the subjects of her impatience, she felt the need to apologize. "I've been unreasonable, bitchy, and emotional. As we go through these ups and downs, don't forget that I love you."

Carolyn reflects afterward: "Challenging health situations take so much out of a person. A caregiver has to do what she has to do, but sometimes other people in her life don't realize the full extent of the stress. I think they need to understand, but they also need to hear that we love them, even if we don't always show them our best selves."

On one of her weekends at home, Carolyn helped Dave with the grand opening of his automated dog wash. It was a magnificent occasion, full of celebration and hope. But the day after the great event, she was racing against time to be at her mother's side before she died. Fortunately, she made it. After her mother's blood pressure rose with elation at her daughter's arrival, Carolyn had the privilege of being with her, holding her hand as she took her last breath. What followed seemed miraculous: the sun cast its rays on her mother's urn, a gold-trimmed flowered lamp, which had been a gift for her parents on their wedding day over fifty years earlier. With that image, Carolyn felt her mother's affirmation. She knew her mother appreciated the care and attention that Carolyn had given her and her mother's two sisters.

Furthermore, she sensed her mother's hand doling out strength to care for Dave in the challenges that awaited them.

The timing of her mother's death seemed providential because soon, ever more sinister symptoms were sneaking up on Dave. First, his right thumb began tingling. Then he complained of cramps in his hands. Before long, he couldn't type or eat with his weakened right arm. Soon, his breathing was heavier, his posture different, his gait slow. And the thuds were more frequent: He fell down the back steps into the snow. He fell out of bed. He fell backward from his stool. He fell forward and rolled onto the floor while retrieving a napkin. He fell mowing the lawn. He fell walking his dogs. Dave explained that the sensation was one of walking downhill, unable to stop himself.

The loathed condition they'd flicked away like a wretched horsefly now seemed to be circling Dave with evil intent. He was eventually forced to give up his pet care business and even his volunteer work at the animal shelter. But Dave was a fighter. He had goals for his life, and he wasn't finished yet. "I'm going to live till I'm eighty-two," he declared, thinking twenty more years might do the job. And then he added with a slight pleading in his voice, "I have to leave a legacy."

In her new role as caregiver, Carolyn was determined to help Dave realize that he had already created his legacy in the countless people he had influenced and mentored. She made it her mission to keep his life as normal as possible and his dreams fulfilled. Yes, she and her husband still had some living to do.

But she also knew, from the lesson she'd learned as her mother's caregiver, that she would need to accept help to achieve her goal.

One of Carolyn's first lessons was to lighten up. She learned to laugh, to see the humor in the unpredictability of their life. She relegated clutter and dirt to the back burner in deference to their needs. She and Dave made a sacred ritual of checking in for evening "briefings"; it was their time to define the life they wanted for the time they had left.

This included travel. They continued to escape to their second home in mystical New Mexico every other weekend. It was healing for both of them and well worth all the packing it took to make their stays doable. But those trips were small potatoes compared to their visit to the Philippines to see sites Dave had known during his military service there. On the way back, they stopped in Hawaii so Dave could catch a glimpse of the memorial at Pearl Harbor. It was the same vacation that saw Dave, with the help of a full-bodied crew, swing across the tree canopy on a zip line.

Carolyn gives her answer to the question posed most often: How do you do it? "Fortunately, his changes came on fairly gradually, so I was able to get good at one challenge before facing the next. For example, driving him around town to all his appointments made me more confident about taking longer drives to our vacation home twice a month, which then convinced me I could handle the Philippines trip."

"That, and help," she continues. "Knowing our time was limited, I really wanted to be Dave's primary caregiver, but I had no illusions about being superwoman. I welcomed the help that was offered."

As it turned out, Dave had one more ambitious trip in him: he wanted to go to a reunion party of fellow politicos in Washington, D.C. By then, his illness had progressed significantly, and Carolyn, thinking this might be his last hurrah, was going to make sure he got there. But this time she didn't even try to do it alone. She enlisted the help of two loyal and capable friends, took a deep breath, and headed for the airport.

The event was everything the couple could have hoped for. Surrounded by admirers from his decades as a political advisor, Dave was showered with accolades. One politician after another attested to the reason for his success: Dave. Stories loped across the room like greyhounds. Stories of the advisor whose integrity could not be compromised. Anecdotes of the man who recognized hidden talent and gave people a chance, launching them into successful and visible careers. Accounts of Dave's mentorship to the young, of the lessons he imparted not only with his words, but through his example.

His glittering legacy.

Dave came home exhausted but exultant. "I'm not going to live to be eighty-two," he announced to Carolyn. "I'm going to live to 102."

Dave lived five more months. He still had a few more goals, one being to publish his memoir, *Goin' to the Dogs*. Another was to renew his wedding vows with the love of his life. He achieved both.

But it was the tender moments with Carolyn that ended his days in tranquility. From his hospital bed in the living room, Dave could awaken to see his wife nearby working her job from home. They would curl up in the narrow bed and watch movies together. She read to him, talked to him, hugged him often.

Carolyn nourished Dave's body and soul as best she knew how, at peace that her husband would die knowing he was loved—and knowing he'd made a difference in the world with a legacy that was more far-reaching than he could ever have imagined.

Del and June

"Seeing her assigned to the care of others enlarged the hole in my heart."

Progressive supranuclear palsy clothed itself in a slow whittling away of activities for June and, in mirrored proportion, for her caretaker-husband, Del. What a full life it had been. The high school sweethearts, born twenty miles apart, Del in a log cabin, June on a ranch, left the confines of small-town mountain living far behind when they married, and filled their years with adventures that took them around the world.

Del's gregarious wife with a face that beamed like a lighthouse was exactly that: his beacon. She supported him while he navigated college, took on the role of caring for their three children as he established his career, hosted all manner of clients and competitors at her creative theme-parties as he climbed the ranks of success in the engineering and business worlds. She steered her husband into bowling, bridge, football, and theater. In turn, she tried out many of Del's pastimes, even the ones she didn't like, such as big-game hunting, rifle shooting, and fishing. But she did share his love of dancing, snorkeling, scuba diving, snow skiing, snowmobiling, waterskiing and most of all, golfing and boating. Add to all that her countless school activities with their sons, and throw in a plethora of cooking, housekeeping, and entertaining at their home, their cabin, their townhouse, and their lake place. As if her life weren't full enough, she saved time to travel to thirty-four countries with Del, as a result of which the couple made friends all over the world. And then there were her local girlfriends, with whom June made, er, mischief. But Del's not talking. "She was a go-getter," is all he'll say. "She had spunk."

So by the time June took her first misstep, caused by the slight dragging of her right foot, she had been completely immersed in the joys of life with Del for over forty years. June herself suspected she might have suffered a mild stroke, but a visit to a neurologist brought the diagnosis of Parkinson's disease. The reality of such a dark prognosis dimming June's light put a hole in Del's heart. If June felt discouraged, though, she didn't show it. "Have I mentioned she was a go-getter?" asks Del. "I'm telling you, nothing could slow her down."

Del had retired four years earlier, so by the time this unnerving diagnosis interrupted their lives, the couple were basking in their robust social circles and active lifestyle. Back and forth between their winter and summer homes, June thrived on all the socializing and physical activity. And they both loved playing golf. But one day on the golf course, June made a disturbing discovery. Even though she had energy enough to walk the green, and even though her swing was stellar, she couldn't summon the power to hit the ball with any force. Eventually, golf became impossible for her.

Another favorite activity was powerboat cruising in their sport yacht. For two months each year, they would sail with several other couples to a chosen destination, most often the Bahamas. As Del's first mate on their fifty-two-foot boat, appropriately named *June Bug*, June performed her tasks brilliantly. But gradually, movement became more difficult and her strength continued to wane. She was forced to turn over the physical aspects of her duties to Del, who would single-hand the boat, or to someone else who would help out.

While June didn't succumb to self-pity, Del wanted more than anything to snuff out the effects of Parkinson's for his wife. He sought out experts, even imploring a Parkinson's specialist to allow June to be a candidate for electronic stimulus brain probes. But unless she had palsy, he found out, the treatment would not be appropriate. She did not, so no luck. The specialist believed she actually had atypical parkinsonism. So for a second opinion, Del searched for the best doctor he could find, and landed in the office of a renowned movement specialist.

The hole in Del's heart enlarged that day when they received a soul-wrenching diagnosis: June had progressive supranuclear palsy, PSP. Advanced. Untreatable. Terminal.

Soon after that pronouncement, the doctor dismissed the couple, saying there was nothing he could do for them. They could find specialists to treat the various symptoms, but the disease was incurable.

Early in their marriage, June and Del had weathered their grief over the stillborn birth of their third son and, many years later, the two had clung to each other when a terrible spinal cord injury from a diving accident rendered their adult son paraplegic, the event Del labeled "the second hole in my heart." And now, though stunned by the news of June's diagnosis and prognosis, Del knew they would get through this together, too. They had so much to live for in the time they had left.

Though the changes had encroached gradually up to that point, they quickly became more pronounced. June started choking on her food, making Del proficient at the Heimlich maneuver. The falls were more frequent. She became dependent on her walker, sometimes even opting for a wheelchair for more security and comfort.

But June just thumbed her nose with bluster at this disease, as surely as she did years before when she stripped off her blouse and bra and plopped herself down at the dinner table to show her husband and young sons how she felt about their showing up to eat wearing no shirts. She'd whipped them into shape, and she would do the same with PSP.

June never slowed down much. She was determined to live as she and Del wanted to live. One memorable trip was the sixty-eight-day *June Bug* voyage from the Florida Gulf Coast to Chesapeake Bay, where the couple visited all the charming little towns along the rivers that fed the bay. Finally, they pulled their boat into Baltimore. Del had his docking duties to think about and he needed to concentrate. "Stay put," he ordered, in the not-really-so-captainish voice he used with his beloved.

"Stay put, stay put, stay put," muttered June in imitation of a three-year-old in the throes of childhood rebellion.

June, after sitting in the bridge with Del for hours, needed a breather. So even though she was wheelchair bound, she didn't stay put. Propelled by her sense of independence, she walked to the stairs that she just knew she could navigate, and started to descend.

Thud.

As she tumbled, she caught the handrail with one arm, destroying her rotator cuff and losing all movement in that arm. Surgery, the doctor warned, would have only a fifty-fifty chance of success, and the therapy would be painful. Did she want it? Her answer was no.

Now that June was confined to her wheelchair, it was hard

to maneuver her onto and off the boat. The height of each dock—and whether it was fixed or floating—were concerns that made Del anxious, and convinced him it was just a matter of time before both he and June would end up in the water. He struggled with the decision, but the clarity of their situation stared him down like a defiant sheriff: it was time to give up the boat. So Del and June left their warm-weather home in the South and returned north to live fulltime among their family.

With that decision, it was time to write the next chapter of their life. But they still had the first volume to sustain them, a tome of comforting memories they could draw on chapter by chapter: golden days on the yacht; hours of snorkeling, waterskiing, and golf; spirited parties and lively dinners. And of course, June's vivacious face glowing in every scene. They were all tucked away in the gilded pages of their story like relics in a baby book.

The man who had always been able to juggle twenty balls at a time was about to discover how challenging fulltime caregiving could be. June now received one hundred percent of Del's attention as her health steadily declined. Her falls became more violent, even with the help of her sturdy U-Step walker. The most dramatic fall required extensive restoration of her mouth and jaws. Her choking increased to the point where the Heimlich maneuver was no longer effective. The doctors urged her to consider a feeding tube, but she would have none of it. So Del began pureeing all her food.

Eventually her walker, at one time a mere prop for all her antics, was replaced with a wheelchair. One of Del's first tasks as a caregiver was to make their home wheelchair accessible. He put a sink in the master bathroom that was high enough for June to roll her chair under; replaced the sunken bathtub with a shower that had no curb to cross; affixed grab rails near the sink, next to the commode, and in the shower; and installed three-foot-wide doors throughout the master suite.

One Easter morning while still in bed, Del was startled by a loud moaning coming from June. He rushed to her side and tried to wake her up, shaking her, talking to her, and sitting her up. No success. She finally regained consciousness after a trip to the emergency room, but Del was distressed by the lack of an explanation for this event. A week later, it happened again. Only this time, the attending physician knew the cause: a urinary tract infection, a common ailment of bedridden patients. Although June appeared comatose on both occasions, she later told Del that she had been aware of everything that was happening, but could not reply. In his distress about the two frightening back-to-back episodes, Del promised himself that he would warn any caregiver he met about UTIs.

Two months later, June aspirated while drinking a malt, landing her in the intensive care unit on a ventilator, pneumonia festering in both lungs. After surviving a torturous week where death seemed intent on snatching her into its talons, June left the ICU. But she wouldn't be going home. Instead, she was taken to a long-term acute care hospital, sporting three new accouterments: a tracheostomy tube, necessary for removing mucus and supplying oxygen; a catheter; and the feeding tube she had fought so long.

Seeing his beloved assigned to the care of others broke Del's heart. It was necessary, he knew, but he also knew that facility would be her place of death. With the help of his family, he kept vigil over his dear wife day after day.

But June was June. She never had been one to give up, and this was no exception. A month after she had been predicted to die, she settled into her new home at a transitional care and rehabilitation center.

For more than two years, June lived each day with the grace she had always possessed. She slept a lot, but awoke to the comforting presence of her husband, who spent at least twelve hours each day in her room tending to the needs that he knew were important to her, as only a devoted husband would know. He made sure her hair was always clean and styled, her skin and lips smooth and moistened, her legs shaven, her dry-eye problem attended to. And he made sure she could hear the voices of close friends and family on speakerphone when they called throughout the day.

Although the tracheostomy tube prevented June from talking with words, Del lived for what she did say: her smile that communicated love, her sigh of contentment, the tongue she stuck out to indicate yes and no, the glint in her eyes that was a beacon to him.

"In my mind," he says, "she came as near to being a saint as anyone I know. I wouldn't have traded this time with her for anything."

And indeed, there he sat, hour after hour, as the sun rose and set, casting its glow on his first mate.

Pam and William

"Our first rule was no self-pity. Instead, trust and obey."

Pam wasn't suspicious when her husband of thirty-four years bought a condominium in Florida and handed over all the financial aspects of the potential investment to her for the first time ever. It would be years before she realized it was actually a gift he would give her, she who knew little about finances.

Nor did she blink an eye when he commented off-handedly that he had developed a minor gait problem while playing tennis. Who would have seen a problem? This was William, who in addition to playing competitive tennis, biked every day and skied often. This was the man who had hiked forty-four 14,000-foot mountains, and together with Pam and the youngest of their five daughters, had built a house—and even some of the furniture in it. A little wobble here and there was understandable.

She wasn't even overly worried when William's internist checked him for memory lapses, voice weakness, and difficulty swallowing. "We'll just keep an eye on him," the doctor had assured her. "Let's monitor him every six months."

Even when the diagnosis of Parkinson's disease came two years later, Pam didn't feel the earth shake. After all, William was still traveling, playing tennis, and hiking. He was also giving back to his community in myriad ways: as church elder, for example, and as a retired city councilman who continued to work on committee after committee.

The physician's plea to Pam to take good care of herself and enlist the help of others rolled right off her back. Not only did she keep pace with her husband, she even added watercolor painting to her schedule. And once she was juried into the art guild, a full calendar of art shows made her busier than ever.

But Pam did take one piece of advice to heart: she kept a

journal, recording her observations of William's symptoms between doctor visits. "It was the most important thing I could have done as it turned out," she says. "I wrote observations, questions for the doctors, and their responses. It's the most accurate record we have of his deteriorating condition."

It wasn't until the uncertain, but terrifying, conclusion that either multiple system atrophy—MSA—or Lewy body disease had slithered into their lives like a venomous snake that Pam fully grasped what William's health decline would mean. Neither one was a pretty prognosis. Indeed, new symptoms were appearing regularly. He now admitted he couldn't balance the checkbook any longer; that would have to be her job. His handwriting was getting smaller and less legible. He was suffering from incontinence. His current minor swallowing problems, his weakening voice, and his slight gait concerns were escalating. As Pam immersed herself in research, she got a glimpse of the reality of the situation: she was now a caregiver to her beloved husband, whose progressive neurological degeneration would eventually escort him to his death.

They were devastated.

The two lay together in bed the day of his diagnosis, hugging and crying as the shadows of nightfall descended upon them, cradling the couple in their darkness. Sadness and fear engulfed them, giving way to anger as the days marched on. At times, the injustice of it all clutched them so tightly it nearly drained the life out of them. *Something like this should never happen to such a vibrant man*, Pam thought.

Gradually, though, Pam and William came to a place of relative peace with a life-changing decision: they vowed to avoid the destructive tyrant of self-pity. They would focus instead on the values they held dear. For William, his compassion, which was so evident in the church and community he served, was even stronger in his home. He understood that his cherished wife was laying down her life for him, and he would do everything in his power to protect and assist her. For Pam, making her husband a priority was a given, and she would devote all her energy to improving the quality of his life. "It's what you do when you love someone," she says. Together, the couple planned to live as fully as they could at every stage of the disease.

With time, Pam learned to balance her care for William with

care for herself, and most importantly, care for their love commitment as a couple.

"William had always been so smart, talented, and self-sufficient," Pam says about her tall, mustachioed husband. "He was humble about his abilities, but I was especially optimistic about his athleticism. I knew his heart wasn't going to give out as the rest of his body declined. In the end, it probably gave him a longer life."

Much of Pam's care for William, therefore, revolved around helping him be as independent as possible for as long as possible in light of his cognitive and physical challenges. Pam notes, "Someone with these diseases can change, sometimes hourly, displaying disturbing physical or mental symptoms. It's so hard to watch." Sensitive to what was going on with William on any given day or week, she filled their time with activities that would stimulate him physically, spiritually, emotionally, and mentally.

It didn't take Pam long to notice that what she did for William's benefit also served to breathe new life into her as well.

Soothing music wafted through the house daily. Travel videos entertained them, even if William nodded off. They would page through his high school and college yearbooks, reviewing the names of his classmates, laughing at the antics he recalled from those years. They pored over family photo albums that chronicled their life together. And many a day found them taking drives to familiar places, to scenic favorites, wherever she and William would find solace. In fact, after William faced the disappointment of being told he could no longer drive, Pam held on to his car—until *he* was ready to give it away.

"My first rule was no self-pity. Once we agreed on that, we were free to really live," recounts Pam. For the couple, putting their trust in God eclipsed any tendency to feel sorry for themselves. "Don't play God; trust and obey" became their daily dose of wisdom. In that way, their primary source of help was God.

Not that it was easy.

Pam's mind vacillated from anguish to serenity and back to distress again; resolve and regret circled around each other. Discouragement was a strong magnet. Pam holds her folded hands to her lips. "I had to live on faith. I prayed really hard."

The immediate answer to her prayers was the people they loved, who offered frequent and unconditional help. Spending time with friends and his church community kept William's mind stimulated. But family held the highest importance to him, so their children flew in as frequently as they could. They had no trouble keeping the conversation going and keeping the smiles alive, which lit William up inside. Nor did family and friends hesitate to take William to restaurants. "People are gracious," says Pam. "We saw so much love and compassion in folks running across the parking lot to help us out, total strangers. We always made sure not to put William in an embarrassing situation. If he didn't feel shame, we didn't have to either. And vice versa: if we weren't self-conscious, he didn't have to be."

Because Pam wanted to be her best for William, she was careful to take care of herself so she wouldn't be a statistic of the "don't bury the caregiver before the patient dies" insight she had received. "I would advise any caregiver to let friends help. Friends are magnificent caregivers, and they really want to help; it's their gift to you." She sings the praises of those who heeded her call to "Just come. The door is always open." She especially appreciated those who, instead of telling her to call if she needed anything, simply told her what they were going to do for her. Some brought food, while others shared magazines and videos with William. Some stayed and talked with him, even when he wasn't able to respond.

Each of those loving gestures was a treasure to Pam and William.

"It's amazing how rejuvenating two hours out of the house can be," Pam says. "I could get so much more done if I didn't bring William along. I would race up the aisles of a supermarket as if on an Indy speedway. I learned I could save time by just asking where things were if I didn't know. And then, if I had time left over, I would go someplace I love, which usually ended up being a park or the library. I would be recharged when I returned to William. It was clear my time away was good for both of us."

Despite her best efforts to stay healthy, however, Pam watched helplessly as rheumatoid arthritis wrapped its grip around her. The chronic autoimmune disease caused her body to mistakenly attack healthy joints, resulting in pain, swelling, and stiffness. Over time, her disease worsened, making even simple, everyday tasks difficult. Yet despite the encroaching symptoms, she continued to take care of most of William's needs, as well as her own.

Now attending to two diseases, Pam underwent a huge shift when she joined a support group for caregivers of patients with progressive neurological diseases. The healing power of other caregivers' companionship—the friendship, bonding, and information—was immeasurable. "We cried and we laughed together. I realized how important it was to be in a group that could find humor. Some groups are focused on complaining. That would send me running, believe me."

It was while she was caring for William in her own weakened state that Pam recognized as never before the value of humor. One of William's engineering friends sent him a joke via e-mail every single day for years. "During that time, I memorized a lot of jokes," she quips. The two also lightened the mood by watching funny movies together. Being *conscious* about staying lighthearted was a habit that cemented itself in Pam, and perhaps did more for erasing self-pity than anything else. It also simply made them feel better.

Regretfully for Pam, she had little choice but to enlist the help of a care center during the last two years of her husband's life because, with her own painful condition, she was physically unable to care for him at home. Nevertheless, she rarely missed a day visiting him there. Every once in a while, she would actually crawl onto his bed—inconveniently twin-sized as it was—and snuggle up next to him, hugging him, and feeling the beauty of their connection.

The final weeks of William's life were lovely beyond measure. Just like she'd always been, Pam was by his side each day, as were two of their daughters, their ministers, and numerous friends. Pam filled her husband's room with classical music and familiar religious songs, and she read Bible verses to him. She bathed him in soothing words about how much he meant to her, and what a wonderful husband and father he was. She reviewed his life with him, reassuring him that he was a man of God, and a gift to mankind.

Pam told William not to worry about her, the girls, or anyone in the family; they would be okay when he was gone. "And, William, I'll be with you in the near future," she whispered.

When the time seemed to be getting close, the hospice nurse made an interesting comment. "You're not going to die today, William," she said as if she possessed some mystical knowledge.

William just rolled his eyes and looked at her as if to say, "Well, duh. I know that. That's why I exercised my whole life."

But the next day, he surrendered to Lewy body disease, as determined by autopsy. A life well lived, a life filled with the care and love of his devoted wife and family, was over.

Fran and Virginia

"Promise me you'll put me into a nursing home when
you can't take care of me any longer."

Alaska was never the same after Fran's seventy-five-year-old
mother, Virginia, left its shores. The entire state was quaking
with reverberations from her laughter; her positive, happy, lively
energy held that kind of power. The river rafting, the hiking, the cruise,
and all the venues they'd visited were infused with Virginia's convivial
humor and dusted with the twinkling in her eyes.

It was a vacation Alaska would never forget.

Even though Virginia's balance issues appeared there for the first
time, they were minor. And even though she bought her first cane on
that cruise, Virginia would appreciate Alaska as a time when she could
still blame her symptoms on something else. Everyone's wobbly on a
ship, right?

The event three years later didn't faze Virginia either, that ordinary
day when she was standing in the kitchen of her West Virginia home. All
she did was turn around when *thud!* She was on the floor. *No problem.* This
had happened a couple of other times over the past two years. *I'll just get
myself on up,* she encouraged herself. Only this time she couldn't. *Well, the
kitchen floor is as good a place as any to do a little problem solving,* she quipped.
Soon Virginia was inching herself across the room in painstakingly slow
movements until finally she reached the telephone. Her niece Terri, who
lived across the street, got the call, and within minutes had let herself in
and lifted Virginia from the floor.

But months later, Virginia had a wake-up call she couldn't ignore.
While driving home from the grocery store with the fixings for a simple
Thanksgiving dinner she was planning for her son and grandchildren,
the car suddenly felt out of her control. Her reactions were too slow; an
accident, she feared, was just waiting to happen. "Dear God," she prayed.

"If you get me home safely, I'll never drive again."

She got home safely. But as it turned out, the accident waiting to happen wasn't out on the street. It was right there in the garage. Virginia reached into the car, brought out the vegetable tray and the fruit tray, carried them both at once to the refrigerator, opened the door, and lost her balance. *Thud*. She banged the right side of her face against the refrigerator and slid down to the cold, concrete floor of the garage. Having closed the garage door after she parked the car, and having adamantly refused Fran's repeated pleas to get the personal safety alarm Life Alert, Virginia was without help. Alone, like the proverbial tree that falls in the forest, there were no human ears that could hear her.

No one knew she was there.

And she was losing body heat by the minute. Straining her eyes to find something in the dark garage she could use to warm herself, Virginia finally spotted a stack of rugs on a table. *You just need to crawl over there*, she told herself. *Slow and easy, like you did last time*. She inched her way to the table. But sadly, when she got there, she had nothing she could grab onto, nor did she have adequate upper-body strength to pull herself up to retrieve the rugs.

It was five hours before anyone found Virginia. Repeated phone calls from her son had led him to call Terri, the relative who lived across the street. But spunky-as-ever Virginia, despite a black eye and a huge bruise where blood had pooled on the right side of her face, fought both an emergency room visit and a suggestion to call her daughter, Fran, and son-in-law, Ken, to let them know what had happened.

She lost both battles. From the hospital, the news traveled to Fran and Ken: even though she had no concussion and nothing showed up on the brain scan, the doctor thought it was highly likely Virginia had Parkinson's disease. She would need to see a neurologist. But Fran had already invited her mother to visit their home in Denver, which the notoriously independent Virginia used as an excuse. "I don't have time to see any neurologist," she informed the hospital staff. "I'm vacationing in Colorado for six weeks."

Indeed, once in Denver, Virginia was content in her expansive basement apartment in Fran and Ken's home, and felt safe in their company. Happy with her new social status as the life of the party among the couple's close friends and among her own friends from church, she was looking forward to vacation time in this setting.

But Fran and Ken saw her visit as an opportunity to get the best help available for the now seventy-nine-year-old Virginia. Her "vacation" would become a tour of medical offices and a six-week voice therapy trial at the university.

Her first medical emergency happened the very first day.

She, Fran, and Ken were lazing around her basement abode, still in their pajamas, laughing and talking. Finally, Fran yawned and looked at her watch. "Well, I suppose noon is a decent time to get dressed," she joked. The three wrapped up their powwow with one final laugh, and the couple went upstairs to start their morning routine. Not ten minutes later, *thud!* Fran and Ken tore back down into the basement, missing a good number of the steps on the way. There, lying on the floor near the kitchen counter, blood flowing from her head, lay Virginia, dazed. They didn't waste a second getting her to the hospital.

Three midnights, a battery of tests, and a neurologist's visit later, Virginia returned home bearing the diagnosis of Parkinson's. Despite no sign of the telltale tremors associated with the disease, some of her symptoms did fit. So the trio settled into life with Parkinson's disease.

After what turned into an extended five-month stay at Fran and Ken's home following Virginia's diagnosis, it was time to return her to her house in the East. With an aching heart, Fran took her mother back to West Virginia and got her settled in. Barely into the house, she looked at her mother—her battle wounds from falling, her slow movement, her blank expression, her waning voice, the pitiful scrawl that was once her gorgeous handwriting—and could not imagine leaving her alone in her home over a thousand miles away. And when she heard her mother's tears and her plaintive question, "Who's going to help me? Tell me what to do," Fran's response was immediate.

"You can't stay here, Mother."

"I know," said Virginia quietly. And with that, they turned around and headed back to Colorado. Virginia left her life in West Virginia— the house her father had built right next to the home where she'd been born, lifelong friends, the dozens of cousins surrounding her, familiar and comforting sights and sounds, her son, another son's widow, and grandchildren all fairly close by. But her new life in Colorado—the land of strong medical facilities and support groups, a daughter and son-in-law who, now retired, were free to attend to her needs, a social life she had already established through church, a comfortable apartment, friends to play cards with, and, of course, Life Alert— brought the promise of a fulfilling new life.

It was a good move.

But good did not always mean easy. It was in Colorado that, after a continued misdiagnosis of Parkinson's disease, Fran and Ken finally found the right diagnostician, a movement disorder specialist, and received the accurate, but dreaded, conclusion: multiple system atrophy, MSA. After researching that little-known disease, Fran finally had an explanation for Virginia's years of falls: orthostatic hypotension, where a sudden drop in blood pressure sends its victim careening toward the floor without notice. She also had an answer to why the Parkinson's medication Sinemet had lost its effectiveness. Now she understood the deterioration in her mother.

Some of the indignities of progressive diseases, such as having to wear adult "diapers," were trying for patient and caregiver alike. Middle-of-the-night calls by intercom meant that Fran had to get up—two or three times a night—to help her mother with her toilet needs. Fran would wait while sometimes her mother went, and sometimes did not. But no matter what, Virginia did not want to lie in wet Depends. After Virginia's next fall, which landed her in the hospital again, Fran sought advice about the nighttime bathroom trials. The doctor suggested catheterization, an idea Fran knew her mother would never accept. But to her surprise, Virginia was willing, and they scheduled the procedure. On the drive home, Virginia turned to Fran and smiled. "Well," she said placidly, "I guess now we can both sleep all night long."

Virginia refused to become a victim to her disease. It was never in her plans, for example, to say no to travel. Fran and Ken, wanting to keep her life as normal as possible for as long as they could, made sure she got around. For as long as Virginia was able, Fran and Ken would load her into the car, and the three of them would laugh their way across the country on their road trips.

Eventually, her disease got the better of Virginia. With time, dissociation, paranoia, and sundown syndrome—the onset of agitation, confusion, and anxiety as the sun sets—brought her to the point where she needed more care than Fran and Ken could provide. With overwhelming sadness, the couple fulfilled the vow to which Virginia had sworn them three years earlier: "Promise me you'll put me into a nursing home—in West Virginia—when you can't take care of me any longer." Not wanting to lose this woman who had so completely wound herself in, around, and through their hearts, they put the decision off as long as they could.

Once again, Virginia gave them a gift. "Yes, I always did say you should tell me when my care becomes too much. But can you find me a place close to you?"

So Fran and Ken would get to see Virginia every day. And that's exactly what they did for the last seven months of her life, after choosing a nursing home near their house that was patient-centered and homelike.

Virginia had a positive attitude by nature, allowing her to accept her prognosis with grace. Having been caregiver to her own mother, and remembering the toll the challenges of dementia had taken on her, she refused to be a burden to her own children. But if you ask Fran and Ken, she was far from burdensome. She was a blessing. Because underneath the physical and mental deterioration that ravaged the family matriarch, they still saw the treasure that was Virginia: her compassion, tenderness, and humor. Pure gold.

Ken and Audrey

"This disease wasn't going to put us away. But we needed support."

There it sat nestled among the weathered copies of *People* and *Good Housekeeping*, a leaflet seemingly calling to him with the words "PSP support group for patients and caregivers." Indeed, it was a beguiling invitation Ken didn't even know he wanted—or needed. Yet he and his daughter, Gen, count the day they saw that flyer in the office of their movement disorder specialist as one of the most important days in their long journey of caregiving.

Ken's wife, Audrey, had been diagnosed with progressive supranuclear palsy by the Mayo Clinic a year prior, and Ken had been scouring the internet for information about where their path might be leading them. Google was okay for finding resources online, but there was something about actually meeting with people who lived the reality— hearing their stories, picking their brains, bathing in their empathy—that was comforting.

"Comforting most of the time, I should say," says Gen. "I have to admit that sometimes I left the meeting depressed. I felt powerless, like I was stumbling down a hill, unable to stop. But really, I don't regret a single meeting I went to. I learned so much about this rare disease."

Ken, as it turned out, was so relieved to learn such groups even existed for such a little-known disease, that he eventually joined two of them. "I was a little confused about why my first group was almost all women," he says. "Statistically, I don't believe all PSP and MSA patients are men. But my second group was just the opposite—almost all men caring for their wives." He wasn't afraid to admit he valued support. With no cure for Audrey, Ken knew he was dealing with something that wasn't going to get better. "If someone has the flu," he reasons, "it's just a matter of time before she'll improve. If an organ gives out, the patient will have surgery and then recover. But this disease, it's a one-way deal. I couldn't have done it without support."

Ken's wife of fifty-five years, and a nurse by training, wanted to be *his* main support, not the other way around, and she tried—all the way to the end. Ken walks over to the collage of photos on the wall. A radiant woman with a smile that flashes warmth and security like a reassuring lighthouse appears in most of them. Audrey was a nursing student when they met, Ken a graduate student studying plant pathology. He was looking for a date to a New Year's Eve party and called the girl he had met only a few times before. The fuse, once lit, flickered along a chain of dates, then erupted into the flame of love that resulted in marriage. The arrivals of children Jef and Gen provided their family all the richness they could want.

Active was the word that best described Audrey. Not only did she work as a nurse, but she also ran every aspect of the family's small home-rental business. Outgoing and ambitious, she headed the PTA, served actively at church, entertained graciously, worked in the yard, and traveled, traveled, traveled. She was a take-charge woman. This was not someone who sat in a rocking chair and watched TV. Ever.

But as Audrey approached age seventy, some of the qualities that defined her began to flicker. Something just wasn't right inside, she complained, and she wondered if she was following the path of her father and several other relatives who had developed dementia at the same age. Her daughter secretly wondered the same thing, describing a couple of conversations with her mother that she labeled "odd." Ken would say she "miscued" in conversation a few times. But testing showed Audrey had no such condition.

Other symptoms cropped up, one after the other like strident dandelions, each of which Ken could explain away with the slightest twist of the mind. Audrey developed carpal tunnel syndrome in both wrists, but of course the stiffness and pain were easily rationalized by all the painting she had done on their rental homes. Her eyes were another problem—infections, dryness, extreme sensitivity to bright light. But then again, she did live in a sunny, semi-arid state.

The tumbles, though, were the most concerning, and harder to dismiss. One day while visiting friends in Arizona, Ken watched in horror as Audrey crashed into the closet of the guest room. It was a hard fall, with no apparent cause. And that spill ushered in many more. On their daily walks, he had to hold her hand because a thud, it seemed, was always lurking around the corner like a heartless bully ready to trip her. Their strolls decreased in length as time went on until finally they had to give them up altogether.

Even though she was bruised and scraped and bloodied and scuffed repeatedly, even though she suffered cranial bumps and black eyes, Audrey, surprisingly, never broke a bone. But that was small consolation for her family.

One day while staying at their winter home in Arizona, the couple took their usual mile-long walk. Without warning, just after they passed through the gate to their community, Audrey lost her balance and toppled, taking Ken down with her. *Bang.* His head cracked on the pavement. Dazed but conscious, he got up slowly and began to help Audrey cross the street to their house. Once there, Ken lay down on the bed.

The next thing he remembered was waking up in the intensive care unit of the hospital—two days later. The story that unfolded stunned the couple's children. It surprised Ken as well; he remembered none of it. Apparently Audrey had noticed her husband was, as she described it, "talking funny." She walked to the phone and dialed 911. When the paramedics arrived, Ken had a seizure, so they flew him to the hospital by helicopter and contacted Ken's daughter. Gen's immediate response was one of panic—not for her father, but for her mother. "Don't leave my mom alone!" she shouted into the phone. "She's unable to walk by herself, and she falls all the time." And with that Gen hung up, baffled at how her mother had handled the emergency with such limited mobility.

The severity of that incident caused Ken to make a tough decision: the couple would move into a senior living facility. And soon, it became clear it was time to explore Audrey's mounting symptoms with a professional. Ken and Audrey's search for an answer was not as circuitous as what many others had experienced. The neurologist they visited cited parkinsonism. A follow-up visit to the Mayo Clinic resulted in a diagnosis of progressive supranuclear palsy.

"For the next year, we were floundering," says Ken. "I didn't know what to do, and advice was hard to find." But finally, the couple landed in the office of a highly recommended movement disorder specialist, who confirmed the diagnosis. He also directed them to a local PSP support group, which Audrey, Ken, and Gen all embraced—Audrey for the company, Ken and Gen for the collective knowledge of the group's lived experience. They were going to need it, they knew.

Audrey's take-charge demeanor was diminishing, while at the same time Ken's was intensifying. With renewed resolve he made a promise to himself: *this disease isn't going to put us away; we're going to be on top of it.* He started by establishing a daily routine that always included getting Audrey out of the house. It was good for both of them.

Their mountain cabin was a frequent destination. Even though Audrey's lack of balance made it difficult for her to negotiate the uneven terrain near the cabin, she still enjoyed the drives up there and the view through the picture window once they were settled in. Exercise classes with the physical therapist were also welcome outings, as were trips to the grocery store and to their children's homes. "I think the reason she was able to keep moving all the way through her deterioration was because, in addition to her physical therapy, we went out every single day," says Ken.

Audrey loved people, so their daily routine often involved spending time with others. Even when she couldn't engage in conversation, she had her own way of communicating. When someone would stop by to say hi, Audrey would take hold of that person's hand—and what a strong grip she had. Like so many people with PSP, she had trouble letting go once she grabbed hold of something, so visitors got a good dose of handholding from their friend. One tender scene happened when Ken took his wife to the hospital to visit one of his former students, for whom Audrey had been a second mother. She loved the young man and showed it by leaning in as if to extend a hug, the two of them clasping each other's hands during the entire visit.

Many people ask Ken how he managed to care for someone with a debilitating disease for such a long time. He just shrugs. He asserts that he learned what to do simply by being around her. "There was no dramatic point at which I said, 'Now I'm a caregiver.' As Audrey became increasingly dependent, I continued to reach out and do more. Of course, she always wanted to help." When one approach didn't work, he looked for another solution. Being quite the handyman, he rigged up the house with grab bars all along the path Audrey took to get around. Memories of his attempts to do the laundry and cooking, though, make him chuckle. "I realized I wasn't a very domesticated man."

So Audrey changed, and Ken adapted. As her voice grew progressively weaker until finally she could no longer speak, Ken developed an intuitive connection with her that often enabled him to understand her when no one else could. Whenever her eyes melted into a glaze, he could still see that flicker of understanding in them as she tracked conversations. When she could no longer smile, he took consolation in seeing her laugh, her whole body shaking for the humor of it all.

But one thing Ken never got used to was Audrey's impulsivity, a characteristic his support group assured him was typical of people with PSP. It was related to degeneration of the frontal lobe of the brain, resulting in impaired executive functioning. But to Ken, it felt like defiance. If he told her to stay put, for example, she would agree, but moments later, she'd be up checking out whatever curiosity, need, or desire had popped into her mind. One day, the entire family descended on their vacation home in order to dismantle it for renters. Of course, since Ken brought Audrey everywhere with him, she got to be part of the whole to-do. And what a frenzy it was. Strong arms heaving furniture back and forth, plucking picture frames off walls, stuffing boxes with knickknacks and valuables alike. The whole family—Ken, Jef, and Gen—was focused on the task of emptying the house.

Meanwhile, no one was watching Audrey. No one.

But why would they need to? Ken had told her to stay put.

Suddenly, *crash!* The trio frantically raced out of various rooms and converged on Audrey, who was standing near a pile of glass that had struck the floor and ricocheted in every direction, inexplicably missing her. The image of the broken picture frame infuriated the family. Hadn't she agreed to stay put? True to her nature, Audrey was just trying to help. But true to her illness, her instructions to remain seated fell victim to the deterioration of several complex cognitive processes, such as modifying her behavior in the light of directives.

Defiance? Not even close. She did finally see her mistake. "I'm sorry. I shouldn't have done that," she said.

Ken grew immensely during his time as Audrey's caregiver. His biggest lesson perhaps was learning to walk in her shoes. Each day, he simply said, "Now I have to do this." Realizing how much giving he had to do each and every day, he developed a mantra that accompanied him at every moment: "I'm living Audrey's life." And with that, he became the kind of caregiver that he would want for himself.

It was only in Audrey's last two months of life, when she was just about out of energy, that Ken encouraged her to lie down and rest. He would turn on music, lie right next to her on the bed, and listen with her for hours.

Audrey died unexpectedly in her sleep, her last attempt, perhaps, to help out.

No complex cognitive processes required.

Letting Go

Daniel and Stephanie
"Please don't let it get too bad. Please."

The crash of the ball against the pins was music to Daniel's ears. Every one of the ten pins toppled and splattered and struck the ground like popcorn in a lidless pan.

Strike.

High fives from Daniel's work buddies flew at him like bats, but the person he really wished would notice his victory was two lanes over. The striking beauty with the lively eyes, stunning smile, and infectious laugh appeared to be the life of the party among her friends. Daniel promised himself he wouldn't let the evening go by without meeting her.

Apparently the salesman was able to sell himself to her that night because Daniel and Stephanie soon became a couple. Seven years later, they married and he became stepdad to her two teenage daughters. The couple made their home a hub for family gatherings and holiday parties, including their annual Halloween bash, Stephanie's favorite. Their gaggle of friends kept their social life alive and, just as he had seen at the bowling alley way back when, Stephanie, always smiling, always laughing, was still the life of the party. Travel sprinkled their agenda, with San Francisco and Hawaii being two of their favorite destinations. And for relaxation, the couple retreated to their rustic mountain cabin, spending their time fixing it up, often inviting friends to join them.

Daniel couldn't have designed a better existence if he had walked into one of Thomas Kinkade's bucolic paintings. Life with Stephanie was idyllic in every way.

But one day, Stephanie came out of the shower sobbing. "Something's wrong with me, Daniel," she cried. "I'm so scared." That wouldn't be the only time she experienced such turmoil. Yet no matter how Daniel asked the questions, Stephanie couldn't pinpoint exactly what was wrong. He had noticed two recent changes in his wife, though. One was that her voice was becoming weaker. The other was that her normally beautiful handwriting was now shaky. But neither had worried him too much.

Then one evening, it became quite worrisome indeed. Stephanie and her younger daughter were cooking together when Daniel heard a scream. He ran into the kitchen to find his stepdaughter with a terrified look in her eyes. There, crumpled on the floor and unconscious, was his wife. When she came to, she was startled and confused.

"We have to get you to the hospital," said Daniel without hesitation. Something was definitely wrong with Stephanie.

And that was the beginning of a long journey of diagnoses and misdiagnoses that would frighten and frustrate the couple as they sought answers to Stephanie's mysterious condition. The first neurologist thought she had Parkinson's disease, the second thought the brain scan signaled multiple sclerosis. A third specialist, this time a movement-disorder authority, concurred with the Parkinson's diagnosis, but allowed a ten percent possibility of a rarer, much more serious condition called multiple system atrophy, or MSA.

Never one to sit still and passively accept adversity, Daniel tried to find more information by attending a Parkinson's support group. It didn't take long, however, to see that Stephanie wasn't following the typical Parkinson's timeline. Her progression was significantly faster and more severe. At the meetings, he had heard about a different group that addressed MSA and another Parkinson's-like illness, progressive supranuclear palsy. This was the first time Daniel had heard the term "parkinsonism," the generic term that describes a category of neurological diseases that affect movement. Without Stephanie's knowledge, Daniel attended a few of the meetings and became convinced his wife had MSA, and when the couple returned to the movement disorder specialist, the doctor concurred. He amended his diagnosis of Parkinson's to MSA.

"When I heard the diagnosis, it was difficult for sure," says Daniel. "But I'm a realist. I thought, well, these are the cards we've been dealt, this is what our future is going to look like, so let's start the journey." Stephanie wasn't so ready to accept this latest diagnosis, though. After all, she'd already "lived with Parkinson's disease" without ever having

Parkinson's. It could be something else, she thought.

More research led the couple to a medical facility in New York for a second opinion. A PET scan determined that Stephanie did indeed have MSA. For Daniel, the long period of not knowing was worse than the diagnosis. Now he just wanted to know how long they had left together.

At that point, Stephanie's symptoms were already making her life challenging, especially when it came to the job she held at a transportation company. Getting to work every day was difficult enough, but putting in long hours was simply no longer possible. So she quit her job. She spent her time researching alternative cures for MSA—enlisting homeopathic practitioners, acupuncturists, and nutritionists, all of whom claimed they could help her. But while those methods did provide occasional, temporary relief of some symptoms, the disease continued to ravage her body. Daniel's heart broke whenever he would see her glancing at herself in the mirror, so saddened by her own appearance. The conversations they had throughout her decline always ended with Stephanie's fervent plea: "Please don't let it get too bad, Daniel. Promise me that." He had no idea what "too bad" would look like, or when it would arrive, but Daniel promised his wife he would do as she said.

A big part of the couple's life revolved around the constant juggling of medications—trying to get the timing and dosages right as Stephanie's symptoms changed and worsened, while doing their best to discern what was working, what was not, and when to return to the doctor as new symptoms arose. The medication Sinemet, for example, had helped Stephanie's movement at first, but eventually lost its effectiveness. An increased dosage, however, resulted in jerkiness.

Because she had so much to consider before leaving home, Stephanie was often reluctant to go out socially. There was the self-consciousness she felt around her erratic movements, but she was also worn out afterward, so making sure she was rested beforehand was essential, as was building in time to recuperate. And, typical of MSA, choking was a concern. "It got old watching the restaurant personnel panic when Stephanie choked, calling in the paramedics with all their shit," says Daniel. "I just did the Heimlich maneuver on her—and I did it countless times."

Sometimes it seemed a lot easier just to stay at home. Nevertheless,

Daniel wanted to do what made Stephanie happy, and he knew how she loved to travel. They did take a few trips, as well as a couple of cruises, which were good times for them. "But, boy, it was such a hard job," he remembers. They grew closer through the disease, and Daniel was grateful for Stephanie's incredible kindness and caring toward him even when she was as sick as could be. She never complained. "It's hard to be a caregiver and husband, and it's just as hard to be a patient and a wife. I hated every minute of the disease, but I wouldn't have traded those times for anything."

Daniel doesn't mince words when he talks about caregiving in the face of such a violent disease, even when the patient was the love of his life. "All the lifting, bathing, changing soiled linens, stopping her choking, getting up multiple times a night. Every single day. All day and all night. For years and years and years." He sighs and shakes his head. "It's unbelievably tough. What drove me to persist was my dad telling me to cowboy up and take care of it. And I knew that as bad as it was, someone always had it worse."

His biggest help came from other caregivers. Daniel feels he would never have made it through Stephanie's illness and death without the camaraderie of the caregivers' support group. "It was comforting and comfortable," he says. "You see that you're not the only one. They understand why you're angry, why you're sad." Group members helped him with advice and resources, but most of all they gave him solace and the perspective he needed to lighten up.

Daniel was another one who learned to just listen for the thud. One day, he was working on his computer at home when he heard a crash. He tore into the kitchen, but not without feeling irritated that Stephanie had failed to use the buzzer to summon him for help. There she was—yet again—lying on the kitchen floor.

"What the hell are you doing?" scolded Daniel.

Stephanie looked up. "Duh, I'm washing the floor," she retorted. He whisked her five-foot, one-inch tininess up off the floor, wondering how in the world wives were able to do the same for their much taller, much heavier husbands.

Daniel continued attending caregiver meetings, where he heard loud and clear how important it was to accept as much help as possible: counseling, support groups, help from friends and family, even antidepressants if needed. Anything helped. "This is no time to be stubborn and try to save the world by yourself," he cautions.

One particularly helpful piece of information for Daniel and Stephanie was that the sooner the caregiver meets with a palliative care team, the better. He paid for a nurse to attend to Stephanie three mornings a week, and he was consoled by all the laughter and joking that went on between the two. It was even more consoling to see that by the time Stephanie's final decline started three years later, the nurse knew her situation so well she could seamlessly support Stephanie's end-of-life needs.

Requesting help from Stephanie's young adult children and other family members had mixed results. "There are often surprises in who is best at helping and who just can't do it," says Daniel. "I don't place any judgment on how people deal with this type of trial." Hospice advised the couple that having family members as caregivers can backfire as emotions get twisted and roles become blurred. Nevertheless, Stephanie was comforted by the presence of her daughters, one of whom spent three days a week with her for three years. But when their mother's deterioration became too emotionally challenging for them, Stephanie replaced her disappointment with compassion and released the girls from their sense of responsibility.

Time moved quickly near the end of Stephanie's life. On New Year's Eve, the couple went out gambling with friends, Daniel holding Stephanie up to the craps table. They both had a great time. But the very next week, she had taken a turn for the worse, as her sickness continued its destructive rampage with renewed vigor. Her daughters came to spend the weekend with her, and she and Daniel had another talk. "She told me all that shit again about moving on after she was gone," he says. "She begged me again not to let it get too bad. I didn't want to listen. It was clear she was just tired of the fight."

By the end of the weekend, he promised her he would call the hospice nurse the following day to talk about the next steps. They had one last talk before bedtime, during which Daniel told Stephanie she didn't have to fight anymore. If it was her time, she could go; he and the girls would be okay.

After that, Stephanie's decline was very, very fast.

The next morning, Stephanie's nurse came over. By then, Stephanie couldn't move her leg—a new development—so Daniel and the nurse lifted her out of the shower, got her dressed and into bed, and the nurse administered morphine.

Several hours later, after the nurse had left, Daniel brought Stephanie to the table, where the two shared bacon and eggs.

Daniel was facing the sink washing dishes, his back to Stephanie, when it happened. He recognized the familiar lack of sound, the giveaway that she was choking. Based on what she had shared in all her previous episodes, Daniel knew she was unaware that she was choking. She was not afraid.

This time, Daniel didn't let it get too bad.

He held his wife tenderly, kissed her on the forehead, and said goodbye. He picked her up, carried her to the couch where he gently laid her, then called hospice.

Andy and Carol

"We love you enough to let you go."

It seemed that by the time Andy had carried her mother through the bumpy ride of parkinsonism, she should have been able to bear the title of principal researcher. Between her medical investigation and the countless doctor and hospital visits, the veteran airline pilot's everyday vocabulary of rudders, radars, and runways was quickly becoming infused with terms like "cognitive changes," "idiopathic," and "end stage."

But "turbulence" was a term that applied to both worlds.

Carol landed in nursing care at age sixty-six—way too young. The thought of her independent mother sequestered in a home with old people repulsed Andy. Based on memories of her grandparents, who looked old, acted old, and talked old, Andy admits she harbored a fear of old folks. But since she was spending all of her days off at the nursing home with her mother, and she had no choice but to sit down with Carol's cronies for dinner and bingo—she quickly gained a new appreciation for the elderly as they shared amazing story after story.

Carol had her own story, and Andy knew it all too well. Five-feet, four inches on a good day, she was a powerhouse: regimented and disciplined, yet gregarious and, as Andy will proudly proclaim, "just a smart ass." Every afternoon, the accomplished, dark-haired nursing professor couldn't wait to cast off her professional wear each day and put on comfort clothes, which for her were a T-shirt and sweatpants. Not for lounging in, mind you, but for capturing the grease and paint splatters from all her handyman work around her house, where she lived alone.

Carol's independence faced its first potential compromise when her doctor discovered an aortic aneurysm. She was in no immediate danger, but her doctor would monitor it to make sure it wasn't growing. Carol had a huge bucket list of adventures, and her medical scare made her realize she wanted to get started sooner rather than later. So she retired early. Her colleagues, students, and family members sent her off with a big splash of celebratory fun befitting her personality.

But the aneurysm wasn't about to cooperate. A year later, Carol was in the hospital undergoing invasive aortic surgery, the aneurysm having grown to a diameter where it had to be repaired. Then, despite her best intentions to recover and move on, Carol had to deal with an infected incision. Six more weeks of daily visits to the clinic to have her dressings changed caused another hiccup in her plans.

By now, Carol was moving slowly and complaining of hip and back pain. *Of course she is*, thought Andy. *She just had major surgery. She'll return to her old self soon.*

But her body would defy her again. At a postsurgical visit, Carol received shocking news: her blood work showed signs of end-stage renal disease. Carol had two choices: dialysis or a kidney transplant. While Carol was exploring the impact of dialysis on her hoped-for postretirement lifestyle, Andy and her brother, Brian, underwent donor testing, discovered they were both a match, and at Andy's insistence, presented *her* kidney as the one that would save her mother's life—no arguments allowed. A month before the scheduled surgery, however, Carol's BUN-to-Creatinine ratio, an indicator of kidney disease, stabilized and rested barely above the level that would warrant a transplant. Much to Andy and Carol's chagrin, there would be no new kidney.

The surgery, infection, countless doctor visits and tests, and now the battle with low kidney function took a toll on Carol. She seemed exceedingly tired and was slurring her speech. Still slow moving, she cited pain. Specifically, she was worried about hip degeneration. But her doctor didn't express concern, so she continued to live at home by herself with frequent visits from her two children.

One evening, after not having seen Carol for a month, Andy invited her to go out for dinner. When Andy arrived, Carol slipped into the bathroom to get ready. Knowing her mom was the furthest thing from "foo-foo" the world had ever seen, Andy didn't even bother to sit down for the two minutes it would probably take her mother to get ready. She looked around the room. Suddenly, confusion jabbed its pincers into Andy's mind.

Something was amiss here.

Bills were stacked on the desk, unpaid. *Mom is meticulous about bookkeeping*, thought Andy. *This is so unlike her*. As she stared at the papers, she was stunned by how tiny her mother's handwriting had become. She looked in the refrigerator. The few items in there were moldy, and it was clear Carol didn't have enough food to live on. Andy peeked in the laundry room, where she could see her mother had not been keeping up with the washing. A flutter of unease taunted Andy. *What's going on here?*

After nearly an hour of knocks on the bathroom door and are-you-okays, Carol finally emerged. At the restaurant, the trip across the parking lot further unnerved Andy. Carol, now walking with a cane, seemed on the verge of falling at every moment. Carol tottered; Andy hovered. Her unease soon turned to alarm.

When they got back home, Andy could hold it in no longer. She burst into tears. "I know there's something wrong with you, Mom," she said, barely able to breathe. "Tell me what's going on." It was only then that Andy learned her mother had been hiding the severity of her condition. She had fallen before—a number of times—but hadn't wanted to worry her children.

"Mom, you can't stay here by yourself. Come live with me or Brian." Andy hesitated to mention the next option, knowing it would distress her fiercely self-sufficient mother, but she had little choice. "Or move into assisted living," she said. "Being alone isn't safe anymore, Mom."

Andy watched her mother's reaction guardedly. Carol lowered her eyelids, and thought for a moment. Then she looked at her daughter and uttered the words that turned Andy's alarm into outright panic. "Well, maybe so," Carol said. Her mother's easy acquiescence convinced Andy something truly was horribly wrong.

The next morning, Andy left on a four-day trip for work. She phoned her mother that evening to check in. No answer. *How odd*, she thought. After several more unanswered calls, Andy dialed her brother, Brian, who went to check on their mother and learned from her neighbors what had happened. The night before, just two hours after Andy had left, Carol had fallen. She'd spent the night on the floor, eventually dragging herself across the carpet to the telephone. Searing from rug burns, she'd managed to dial 911.

Carol spent ten days in the hospital, where testing revealed a low white blood cell count, but not much else. However, on one of Andy's frequent visits, the rehabilitation doctor approached her. He had just completed an assessment of Carol, and he had one question for Andy. "Does your mother have Parkinson's disease?" he asked.

"No," said Andy, her bottled-up fear breaking through with force. "Why are you asking that?"

"Her flat affect is symptomatic of Parkinson's," he said, adding, "along with many of the other symptoms you've seen in her."

Forty-five days in a skilled nursing facility followed. Practice walking, sitting, and standing would build strength, but Carol would never go home again. Instead, she moved into assisted living, where all her hours with a physical therapist couldn't help her gait issues. Even with the walker, Carol had trouble moving her legs, often rocking back and forth up to forty times before she could lurch forward, and then only when someone tapped her leg to get it going. She also suffered many falls.

Although the disease did not affect her memory, Carol did show cognitive changes. Multitasking was nearly impossible, for example, and her ability to reason was declining rapidly. Dialogue was limited, less detailed, and her smarty-pants attitude was mellowing.

But the hallmark Parkinson's tremors were never present. So finally, Andy and Brian took their mother to see a neurologist. A lack of response to dopamine-replacement Sinemet eliminated Parkinson's disease. Since no laboratory or brain scan testing existed for any specific atypical parkinsonism, the best the doctor could provide was a clinical diagnosis of a neurodegenerative disease, which could have meant progressive supranuclear palsy, multiple system atrophy, the even rarer corticobasal degeneration, or Lewy body disease, among others.

"I'll say she has MSA," the neurologist finally ventured. "But it doesn't really matter. Simply put, your mother's life span will be short, she'll need care, and there's no cure."

Carol eventually left her assisted living apartment—where the staff had found her many times on the floor, having rolled off the couch— and returned permanently to the skilled nursing facility. While follow-up testing eliminated the presence of Alzheimer's disease, the frontotemporal dementia she did suffer from would insure further mental decline. Hardly any consolation.

That's when Andy became an avid researcher. The neurologist gave her a thick book on parkinsonism, which she read cover to cover. Through her reading, Andy learned of the cognitive issues to come, specifically difficulties with those functions controlled by the brain's frontal and temporal lobes: planning and judgment, emotions, speaking, understanding speech, and certain types of movement. She also made it a point to learn how to support her mother as her physical condition declined.

During Carol's two-year stay at the nursing home, she ended up in the hospital on several occasions. After one weeklong stay, a kidney biopsy showed she'd had cholesterol crystal embolism. The nephrologist went on to explain that cholesterol crystal showering can occur spontaneously or as a result of invasive surgery. The latter, he believed, was the cause of her kidney disease. But because she was terminally ill, she still would not be a candidate for a kidney transplant. With that, Andy stepped resolutely into the role of Carol's primary healthcare advocate.

Andy knew the process of letting her mother go had begun. She made it her job to insure that Carol's life was happy. Knowing how it must have pained her mother not to be able to continue the habit of reading her usual five-to-seven books per week, Andy would read to her short sections from *Reader's Digest* or the newspaper. She helped her mother solve her beloved word jumbles, scrambling to jot the words down as fast as her mother solved them. They watched TV together until the day came when Carol lost interest.

Andy also made sure her mother was safe each day. With Carol's more frequent falls, she now sported a soft-sided helmet to protect her head. She hated it, of course, but because she had a front-loaded gait, with her head leading her walk, a thud was always imminent. To increase safety, the chaise lounge shape of her wheelchair prevented her from getting up and tumbling to the floor. Her new bed was equally novel: shaped like a shell or a shallow cup, it prevented Carol from rolling out while still allowing her to sit up and look around.

When Carol announced one day that she had been talking to her mother, who had been dead for years, Andy recognized this phenomenon as a sign that death was near. She began to prepare herself for the inevitable.

On the day Carol passed away, fear of the not-yet-known circled in and out of certainty that all would be well. With the doctor's prediction that their mother had anywhere from one hour to three days to live, Andy and Brian phoned relatives. "If you want to say goodbye, you'll need to come *now*," they said. Family arrived, filtering in throughout the day. After the last relative arrived, Andy knew her mother would be leaving them soon. She and her brother moved their chairs right up to her bed and rested their heads tenderly on her shoulder. Trusting she could hear them in her comatose state, they spoke the words they knew she needed to hear: "We love you enough to let you go, Mom."

Within mere hours, Carol, surrounded by family, took her final breath. To Andy's great relief, Carol's passing was as gentle as a skilled descent through soft clouds followed by a flawless landing.

The lighthearted mom may have physically left this earth, but she certainly had the last word: her legacy of love, laughter, inspiration—and yes, cheekiness—is firmly rooted in her offspring.

Ruth and Jim

"Our life was full of serendipity."

Serendipity made a habit of showing up throughout Ruth's life. Going steady with Jim in high school, being his prom date, wearing his ring, boating their summer days away, and watching him as a roper in rodeos—all were the first sturdy strands of their cosmic net.

But graduation signaled the end of their relationship, she seeking a career out of state in deaf education, he staying in town where he eventually started his own trucking company. Their paths crossed only occasionally at first, then never.

Until thirty years later when fate reared its head.

Jim was newly single and often thought about Ruth, who was, in his words, "the woman I'd loved all my life." A quick phone call to Ruth's sister sent him on a quest to New Mexico, where Ruth was teaching at the university. "That was the beginning of a great renewed romance," muses Ruth. They married three years later.

One day, on the way back to their house, the couple decided to swing by a lake where they happened upon three different marinas, each with its own charm. The draw of the water was irresistible, and that serendipitous detour led them to buy a boat. Through their weekends on the lake, they gathered a circle of friends called "Boats in the 'Hood," who would join them for extended stays on Lake Powell and Lake Meade.

Those trips awakened something deep inside Ruth. Not only did memories of their boating as teenagers surface, but her own parents' lifelong, yet unrealized, desire to live on a boat titillated her. Within a short period of time, Jim and Ruth had bought a yacht, let go of their work responsibilities, and moved to Texas to find a slip for their new home.

Once in Texas, another surprise awaited Ruth. As her interview for a teaching position was about to begin, she was startled by the interviewer's initial comment: "I know you." Ruth soon realized her soon-to-be superior had been her intern in another state over thirty years earlier. A new job now secured, Ruth turned to the challenge of finding someone to sponsor them in the marina. Again, Ruth was on the receiving end of good fortune when her new boss said, "Yes, I know someone who will sponsor you."

With everything falling together so providentially, it looked like Jim and Ruth had achieved their dream. They were together at last, deeply in love, and living on the sea.

This was the life Ruth had dreamed of. But in writing her script, she had never imagined the role of "caregiver." She and Jim had places to go.

The couple had one more current of their dream to pacify: they wanted to circumnavigate eastern North America by water, on a cruise called The Great Loop. The Intracoastal Waterway, a three-thousand-mile trek along the Gulf and Atlantic coasts, would also lead them inland through rivers and across lakes. But that trip would have to wait until Ruth retired for good.

While Ruth was fulfilling her new teaching position, Jim stayed home, where he would help their marina neighbors work on their boats, painting and doing repairs for them. One day, he was reaching for a light bulb when suddenly he fell off the ladder. After the initial shock, he was disturbed that he couldn't right himself. A short while later, he was riding his bike when, again, he simply tipped over—for no apparent reason. He ended up with a torn rotator cuff that time, the first of many injuries that would compound over the next few years: bruises and scrapes and hard knocks on the head, a shoulder that wouldn't heal, chronic neck pain, a pinched nerve, a gash over his eye, a second torn rotator cuff, knees that were bone on bone. It was one injury after the other, with no healing before the next affliction befell him.

Little by little, Ruth was stepping into her new role.

One night, Jim couldn't breathe. Terrified, Ruth took him to the emergency room, where the consensus was that this frightening episode was due to his not wearing a mask while painting inside the boat. From that day on, Jim blamed every symptom that emerged on toxic paint fumes. He continued falling off his bike—an effect of toxic paint fumes. He succumbed to his lack of balance when it got windy—toxic paint fumes. His eyes didn't track—those fumes again.

After five years living on the boat, Ruth was finally able to retire. Amidst all of Jim's medical emergencies, the couple still held out hope of spending a year navigating The Great Loop. Ruth wasn't going to let Jim's health issues slow him down; she would be there to help him. She also knew how important it was to think of her own self-care. "I was learning that if I wanted to keep my life interesting, I had to keep his life interesting; what was good for him was good for me," she says.

But a month before their departure, the two were rear-ended while driving home, ironically, from Ruth's retirement luncheon. Though Jim was hurt—he tore his rotator cuff again— they sought exercises instead of surgery this time. Serendipity had struck again: if they had gone through with surgery and had to wait five months to begin their journey, they would never have started their cruise.

At last, in June, Ruth and Jim embarked on The Great Loop. They were in Mobile, Alabama, heading to Jacksonville, Florida, when they got wind of a hurricane heading their way. The warning prompted them to head north to Demopolis, Mississippi, and wait out the storm. That tempest grew into Hurricane Katrina, which, as history would later reveal, caused widespread devastation. Even though Jim and Ruth were spared its immediate effects, they were detained when pleasure vehicles were banned from the waters as FEMA did its work getting supplies to damaged areas.

And then the couple got caught in one of life's eddies that stalled their plans. As they were waiting for post-Katrina life to return to normal and allow them to launch The Great Loop again, Jim pulled out his fold-up bicycle and passed his time riding. One day, he lost his balance and fell, as he had before. A chiropractor was their specialist of choice this time, but the doctor could see chiropractic was not the solution. "I'm not going to treat you," he said. "I think you have a pinched nerve, and I'd like you to see a neurologist." They returned to Houston, leaving their boat in Demopolis. A flood of surgeries began—four in nine months—which brought their travel plans to a grinding halt.

The serendipity in this long journey of mysterious symptoms, surgeries, and more thuds than they cared to count was not that it led to the correct diagnosis. Clearly, it didn't. For seemingly isolated symptoms, Jim had seen many specialists throughout the years, each one patching up only what fell into his or her area of expertise: chiropractor, ophthalmologist, orthopedist, various surgeons, cardiologist, physical therapist, neurologist. The neurologist thought he had found the missing link to Jim's symptoms. He noted shaky handwriting that pointed to Parkinson's disease, cognitive issues that resembled Alzheimer's, but finally pulled it all together with a diagnosis of traumatic brain injury due to anoxia—depletion of oxygen from having so many surgeries so close together. But he, too, was wrong.

No, the serendipity of their lost dream was that it led the couple on a different loop—full circle back to where they had met as teenagers. With The Great Loop adventure out of the picture, the couple, though heartbroken, made the decision to return to their hometown, far from the sea and their comfortable life on the yacht. While Jim continued his various therapies, it was back home where serendipity sided with them once again, this time to tie his symptoms together into a correct diagnosis.

A neurologist affiliated with a renowned brain injury center in a nearby university town made the most definitive statement yet. "Jim's been misdiagnosed," he averred. "He has either progressive supranuclear palsy or multiple system atrophy. Since you've witnessed all of his symptoms over the years, I'm going to ask you to look up these two diseases on the internet and tell me which one fits Jim better." Ruth immediately identified Jim's symptoms as compatible with PSP. The doctor sent all of Jim's records to the prominent movement disorder specialist in the area, whose pronouncement confirmed Ruth's worst fears: "Jim has advanced progressive supranuclear palsy."

The days ahead were dark ones for Jim and Ruth. From her research, Ruth knew that Jim's disease was not a pretty picture and that the love of her life would be leaving her long before his time. "The diagnosis changed my view. I always thought that if we just worked hard enough, we could defeat anything. Now we had a disease that was going to defeat us," she says. For a couple who had defined their ideal life and taken gutsy steps to make it happen, this was a hard blow, and the powerlessness was crushing.

Jim never became hostile, but the two cried together often. One day, Jim tried to describe how he felt. "It feels like my mind is in a cocoon," he said, and Ruth thought her heart would break. His intelligence was alive, but it was trapped inside by his rapidly decreasing ability to express himself. And his body refused to cooperate, too. He was aching to pedal a bike or launch a boat. He yearned to explore more of the world, but his walls were closing in. Through yes and no squeezes, now his only language, he was able to receive the life-prolonging treatments that he wanted, refuse those he didn't want, and receive visits from close family and friends.

A severe choking incident from which Jim never recovered finally took his life. In the end, he died at home, the woman he had always loved by his side, as she had been through all their adventures.

It was the final serendipity that made it easier for Ruth to let go. Apparently, the night before he died, Jim's spirit took sail and circled around to each of his grandchildren. One son reported that his wife saw Jim standing in the baby's room, "as real as he is real." And Jim's other son knew exactly to whom his young daughter was talking when he heard her say on the intercom, "Good night. I love you, too."

For Ruth and Jim, their Great Loop was now complete. But he wasn't far away.

PART 2
LAUGHING

Falling Free

The golden aspens flickered outside the window of the living room. Daniel was inside, reflecting on his life with Stephanie, his wife of way too few years. He still held disdain for the horrendous disease that had robbed her of her independence, robbed him of the love of his life, and robbed them both of the dream life they had envisioned together. The news that she would decline until her death had left Daniel feeling isolated.

Until he discovered a caregivers' support group.

"I could never have gotten through this journey without the group," says Daniel. "It's essential that people not try to go this alone."

Daniel even led the support group for three years. Just as the members had provided friendship when he felt alone, he, too, reciprocated when he could, and over the years he had made several close friends.

One of those friends was Joe.

Joe was well into his decline when Daniel befriended him and his wife, Helenn. When the two men spent time together, they would usually just take in a movie or share a beer at a bar. He also took his friend golfing—Daniel would just prop Joe up next to the cart and let him swing at the ball.

When Joe was with Daniel, he was a pro.

One day, Daniel decided he knew exactly what Joe needed: to be exposed to some of the dangers from which his wife constantly protected him. He needed some excitement. And Daniel knew he was just the person to provide it.

So he waited until they were well out of range of Helenn's hearing, then proposed his idea.

"Let's go skydiving, Joe."

It took no convincing. Off they went to the indoor skydiving facility, where gigantic fans in the vertical "flight chamber" simulated the real experience. The airflow was strong enough to keep a person hovering above the ground for a few exciting minutes.

In preparation for their "flight," Daniel read the list of restrictions. "Hey, Joe. We got a few rules to read. Help me out here. Are you under three years old?"

Thumbs down.

"Pregnant?"

Thumbs up.

"Very funny, Joe. Any prior shoulder dislocations?"

Thumbs down.

"Back or neck problems? In a hard cast? You over 250 pounds?"

He fired off the rules one after the other like BBs on a target. Joe had no limitations.

"Okay, buddy, we're good to go." Daniel suited him up, placed his goggles securely over his face, fastened his helmet, helped him insert the earplugs—and let him fly. He watched his friend, splayed against the wind, flight suit flapping as he floated on a column of air.

Three minutes of complete and utter freedom.

When he brought Joe home, Helenn asked where they'd gone. Daniel kept mum.

When Joe left the house with Daniel, he was all-powerful.

Enough said.

Ado in Honolulu

As an airline employee, Carolyn was a seasoned traveler. Standby traveler, that is. She'd been back and forth between her home and her mother's and aunts' homes every other weekend as she cared for them in their declines. But now they had passed away, and she could devote all of her caregiving to her husband, Dave. Given his terminal illness diagnosis, she wanted to support him in achieving his dreams.

So why was she surprised when he asked to go back to the Philippines where he'd served his military duty? Fact was, he didn't just ask; he said he was going with or without her.

She figured she'd better pack her bags.

Planning a trip for standby travelers could be challenging, but Carolyn had access to all the information she needed to determine their best chances of getting on board a flight. Sometimes they had to be creative, as when flights were full, but she'd become a pro at choosing alternate routes at the last minute. In the many years she'd been doing this, they'd always managed to get to their destination one way or the other.

The first leg of their trip landed them in Honolulu, where they would spend the night. *Might as well make the best of being in a great location overnight*, thought Carolyn. The following morning, they would visit Pearl Harbor, but they had a whole evening in front of them. What should they do?

Carolyn suggested taking a walk, preferably to the row of shops across the street. The *six-lane* street. Dave was game, so they secured a wheelchair from the hotel and set out to take in the sights. Sure, Carolyn had never navigated Dave in a wheelchair, but she'd seen people do it. How hard could it be?

"Ready? I'm running us across the street. Hang on!"

She glanced right and then left, and then thrust Dave and his chair into the empty street. Pushing as fast as she could, she checked for cars one more time halfway across. None in sight. More confident now, she picked up her pace and trotted across the pavement like the fabled hare bolting off the starting line. Then with no warning whatsoever, *thud!* Dave catapulted out of his wheelchair and landed flat in the middle of the street. The chair had hit a crack in the road.

Carolyn was aghast.

And then the two burst into laughter simultaneously.

Onlookers witnessed a terrifying sight, but Dave and Carolyn were snorting and chortling in hysterics—so hard, in fact, that she couldn't pick him up. Within seconds, two Good Samaritans screeched their car to a halt and sprinted toward the scene. It took nothing for them to rescue Dave and get him upright in his chair.

"Don't you know how to push a wheelchair?" the driver scolded Carolyn before returning to his car.

"Well, no, as a matter of fact. This is my first time," she said.

"It's like a baby stroller—you have to back the thing up when there are cracks and then ease over them," the other admonished as he closed the door and the two sped off.

"But what if I didn't see the—" Carolyn protested, only to realize she was talking to a trail of exhaust.

Laughter followed the couple as they continued their trek across the street. When they reached the curb, Carolyn lifted the wheelchair back—like a baby's stroller.

"I think I'm getting the hang of this," she gloated.

And they laughed their way through the evening, making a good time out of a close call.

The Last Word

Myriad words described Carol. "MSA patient" was her family's least favorite. However, portray Carol like she was—smart, gregarious, self-sufficient, positive, authentic—and the picture becomes clearer. She was all that. But nothing fit Carol better than her daughter Andy's favorite tag: smart ass.

By the time Carol was receiving palliative care, a rare neurodegenerative disease had whittled away almost all of her motor skills. Perhaps most difficult for her caregiver children, Andy and Brian, was her inability to speak. They knew she could understand them, and they spoke to her often, but they longed for a return to the days when they could soak in her experience and wisdom, her playfulness, and her obvious caring, through dialogue. Sadly, that was not to be.

One day, the palliative care team came to evaluate Carol. Their goals were to formulate a plan of care, to let Andy and Brian know how to keep their mother comfortable, and to address any family issues so that everyone was on the same page for Carol.

But something was missing: Carol's input.

"Do me a favor, Brian," the doctor finally said. "Let's talk to your mom and see if there's any response." He directed Brian to ask a simple yes-or-no question. Brian walked to his mother's side and stared into her open, but blank, eyes. She immediately tracked her stare to him.

"Can I ask you a question, Mom?" Brian sounded tentative.

No answer from Carol.

Brian cleared his throat. "How are—" No, he had to make sure his mother could answer with a yes or no.

He started over. "Are you fine, Mom?"

Again no response.

He tried again. "Are you fine, Mom?"

Her gaze was focused squarely on her son, but no response came.

He tried tweaking his question slightly. Maybe using her name first would catch her attention. "Mom, are you fine?"

Silence.

The group exchanged glances. The doctor scribbled notes.

Then, off-handedly, Brian asked, "Want me to shut up?"

"YES!" The word flew out of her mouth like a suppressed howitzer just waiting for its turn.

It was the last time she would speak. At that moment, Carol closed her eyes and never opened them again.

Yes, she did have the final word.

Smart ass.

The Potato Dance

With each attempt to brighten Lee's days, his wife, Callae, and daughter, Deri, learned to see the light side. In the midst of sadness, they discovered humor. It saved them from utter anguish and hopelessness, and snowballed into a habit of lightheartedness.

Take the potato dance, for example. Callae always wore jeans with back pockets, and she wore them for good reason. When she helped Lee walk, he would face her and put his hands in those pockets while she put her arms around him and grabbed onto his gait belt. Then together they would hobble to their destination.

Friends would tease them about this technique, which they called "Callae and Lee's potato dance"—likening it to the party game where participants pass a potato under their chins, one to the next, until someone drops it. Except that Callae and Lee *were* the potatoes. They were so in sync, in fact, that when Lee fell, he did so gently, and Callae would often float right down with him. It was as graceful as a ballet.

They'd just laugh. And laugh some more.

And then there was the ski jump.

Lee's mind moved faster than his feet. One evening, after a discouraging day of slow movement, he decided to take a walk around the living room. At one point, the front of his walker was a ways out in front of him, but his feet were still planted in place on the floor, giving the impression of a skier launching off a jump. Deri told him as much. "Dad, you look like you're ready for the Olympic ski team!"

A wide smile spread across Lee's face.

For so long, Lee had regretted that Callae and Deri had to suffer right along with him. But with Deri's joke, he lightened up, no doubt relieved that his family could laugh with him at times.

That was Lee, still wanting to protect those he loved.

Limbo Like Me

June, with her love of people, her creativity, and her instinct for making everyone feel welcome, had hosted countless galas. "It was a huge loss for her when her physical condition worsened," says her husband, Del. "No more parties to plan. It had been such a big part of her life." So when June and Del joined a boating community, they were ecstatic to see that their nautical friends were equally fun loving. In fact, the boat owners took turns planning activities for the entire group.

One such festivity was a Limbo party with a Gilligan's Island theme. The Limbo was a dance from the 1960s, in which participants hopped under a horizontal bar that got lower with each round. By the end, the winner was the one who could contort his or her body—like the childhood toy, Gumby—far enough backward to clear the pole. Obviously, good balance, strong ankle and leg muscles, and a healthy ego were assets. June had none of those except the healthy ego, bolstered by a strong sense of fun.

The guests arrived ready to party. Palms decorated the walls, lawn chairs abounded, and colorful rum drinks coated the throats of one and all. Some of the men, bedecked in screaming-bright leis draped around their necks or over their heads like crowns, flaunted their grass skirts and one-size-fits-all coconut bras. Everyone else just wore tropical shirts, except for June, who dressed as Gilligan—jeans, red knit shirt, white sailor cap sitting askew on her head, gigantic costume sunglasses keeping their balance on her nose.

Suddenly the lyrics of Chubby Checker, "Limbo, limbo, limbo like me," invited dancers to the floor. "Ohhhhhhh, limbo like me!"

June was ready. This was her opportunity to show that no disease would hold her back. She zoomed her wheelchair right over to the pole. One of the captains served as her partner, and together those two cleared the horizontal bar inch by inch as it was lowered round after round. When the last dancer remained, no one was surprised to see it was June, pumping her arm in victory, her eyes sparkling, her face gleaming with the pure joy of it all.

Take that, Limbo stick.

Cruisin'

As Phil's condition worsened, he and his wife, Barb, continued to hold firm to their vow to live life fully. They had always been hardy travelers, so they thought nothing of taking the family on an Alaskan cruise—right after a weekend of partying in Monterrey, California, where they would be celebrating a family friend's wedding.

Let's just say they stayed out a bit too late and danced a little too hard at that wedding reception.

And boy, did Phil's body object, punishing him with a painful, sleepless night. Barb was right by his side, wide awake. So by the time the family landed in Anchorage the next day for the cruise, Barb felt like she was eighty years old. Forget pride. She arranged for a wheelchair for Phil, his first ever.

But it wasn't she who pushed him.

There, right next to Phil, trying heroically to keep up with him, was Barb—in her own wheelchair. Their adult children were mortified. But, as the couple's limited energy reserves quickly burned out, the children took over. The Anchorage airport got an eyeful with the foursome gliding across the glossy floor, two wheelchairs and two weeks' worth of luggage—but not a trace of discouragement on anyone's face.

The folly continued when they discovered—the hard way—that the seven-tiered cruise ship was not wheelchair accessible. In the Alaskan rain and sleet, Barb and her son strained to push Phil up the gangplank, as throngs of impatient passengers followed—right behind them.

With the nearly superhuman energy of Olympians, they kept the chair going, up, up, up, stopping occasionally to let people pass them, but never daring to let go of their grip, not even for a second.

"We could've wiped out the whole ship if he had slid back," said Barb soberly.

Phil feigned a grimace, then laughed. "Aw, a little life-threatening experience like that didn't ruin our fun," he said. "It was worth it."

Sass

R eceiving the diagnosis of a terminal illness was not the trajectory
Annette and Mike had envisioned for their marriage. While Mike
presented apathy in the face of his deterioration, but never with
anything more negative than "I wish this weren't happening," Annette
adopted a different stance.

"This was our life. This was how it was going to be, and it wasn't
going to change," she says. "I had no choice but to find the positive in our
day-to-day life."

So she had mixed feelings toward the suggestion that she and
Mike join support groups—she for caregivers, he for patients who were
also suffering from the same disease. Annette dreaded the thought of
being dragged down by a room full of caregivers droning on and on about
their woe-is-me lives. Self-pity bored her at best; at worst, it just plain
irked her. But after further consideration, she eventually caved. She would
do it, but she would have none of that moaning and groaning. After all,
if her fellow caregivers couldn't appreciate her "incidents" with Mike, no
one could. She planned to share them all with her group.

And that she did. As might be expected, caregiver support
meetings were always a party when Annette was there.

Take the story she told, for example, about all the stains on the
carpet anywhere and everywhere a dog—or an incontinent person—
might go. Annette never knew if she was cleaning up after her canine or
her husband. But even more confused was the dog. Why, he seemed to
ask, can't I "go" inside like Mike does? Annette threw up her hands. All
that doggy training, down the drain.

Sometimes Annette witnessed Mike's shenanigans herself; other
times, she only *heard* about them after returning from an afternoon of
errands. Even though she was his primary caregiver, she wasn't averse to

bringing healthcare aides into their home for increasing amounts of time as his illness progressed. Nor was she afraid to admit she needed to take a break. One year, she was even able to fly off to a vacation resort in Florida while Mike went to "summer camp" at a nursing home.

Truth was, Mike was in his element while Annette was gone. He loved all the attention he got—from the physical and occupational therapists, the young female aides, and the friends Annette had arranged to visit him. The older ladies, of course, had the most life experience, and Annette herself favored them, especially the one she secretly referred to as Martha Stewart—because of her expertise in folding those infernal fitted sheets. While Mike was always a gentleman, he rather preferred the woman with the beautiful, flowing hair that she would toss jauntily as she sauntered around the room. Or the one who had a, shall we say, *generous* chest—Mike tended to find extra things he needed her help with.

Annette always got reports from the visiting nurses and aides when she got home. It was after her rare vacation trip that she got wind of Mike's nightly whimpering: "Who's going to tuck me in tonight?"

Remembering, she rolls her eyes.

"And then there was the time the evening homecare aide reported Mike's sassiness," she says.

Seems Mike had been eating with his hands, as he usually did once his ability to manipulate silverware began to decline. The conscientious aide figured she'd better do something about his mucky hands and food-loaded fingernails. So she set out a bowl and filled it with boiling water, let it cool somewhat, then lifted Mike's hands and immersed them. According to her report, Mike quickly pulled his "burning" hands out of the tepid water.

"What are you using me for, soup bone?" he protested, pretending to be horrified.

Mission Accomplished

One day in early November, Barbara watched Jerry stare at the TV for hours. *Not good*, she thought. *This man needs a project.* She broke his trance with a proposition.

"How about we do something fun?" She spelled out a plan she'd been thinking about for a while.

What would Jerry think about transforming his stunning nature photographs into cards? The accomplished photographer had already done the work, long before his illness had taken its toll. Barbara would write thinking-of-you sentiments on each one. And then the best part: they would sneak down the hallways of their apartment building—late at night, of course, to pump a whodunit element into the scenario—and tape a card onto each of their neighbors' doors.

"What do you think, Jer?" Barbara looked past the expressionless mask brought on by his neurological disease, no smile betraying his enthusiasm for the project. But she found what she was looking for: that twinkle in his eye.

"I'm in," he said.

Together the couple pored over the many striking photos Jerry had captured over the years. Each one brought back a memory—not only of the place it was taken, but of what they were doing, words spoken, feelings felt, and dreams dreamt at that time.

Once they decided on the pictures they would use, they fired up the computer, and it wasn't long before Jerry had imported all his photos: mountains, canyons, waterscapes, sailboats, bouquets, sunsets, and gardens, all chock-a-block on the computer screen. Barbara printed the photos on card stock, then cut and folded 50 two-inch-square cards—enough to greet each of the building's residents. The biggest challenge was finding varied ways to say "thinking of you," but Barbara managed to come up with them.

By the week before Thanksgiving, their gifts were ready to deliver.

At zero dark thirty on the night of the secret mission, Barbara quietly opened the door and peeked out, her eyes sweeping back, then forth, then back again. "Coast is clear," she whispered. While Jerry held the basket brimming with colorful shards of paper on his lap, Barbara pushed the wheelchair down the top-floor hallway of the four-story apartment building. Suddenly a door cracked open and voices leaked into the hallway. With the stealth of a seasoned spy, Barbara maneuvered the wheelchair into a dark recess, where she and Jerry hid until the voices faded. A few tense moments later, they emerged.

The couple headed toward the farthest apartment and, pausing at each alcove, Barbara reached into the basket and furtively affixed a card to the door. As they neared the elevator, they heard it cranking upward in their direction. *Oh-oh.* On the run again. Barbara and Jerry tore down the hall and around the corner, barely managing to avoid detection.

Once their work was done on the fourth floor, the couple rolled innocently back to the elevator to begin the assault on the rest of the building.

By the time they reached the main floor, the contents of the basket were shrinking. With more traffic here than on the other three floors due to the comings and goings at the building's entrance, the couple were forced to halt the operation several times.

"Diversions!" Barbara hissed. "We need diversions." So Jerry reached down to pat the ears of a passing dog, deflecting attention to the friendly little animal. They stopped to converse with a couple, who didn't even notice the basket. They dipped into the darkened kitchen momentarily while several more people strolled through the front door. Finally the home stretch was in view. Forty-eight, forty-nine, fifty. The basket was now empty. They darted back to their own apartment, threw open the door, and slipped in.

Mission accomplished.

For Jerry, their caper was a shot in the arm. He fell asleep that night knowing he had made people happy, had shared his gift of photography, and had just plain had fun with his wife. The appreciative comments from their neighbors spurred Jerry and Barbara to repeat their quest at Christmas, and again with poems at New Year's. While preparing Valentine's cards, Barbara looked over at Jerry.

"This is becoming addictive!" she confessed.

Road Trip Feat

Fran and her husband, Ken, loved road trips. So did Fran's mother, Virginia. She was an enthusiastic traveler and ready for any adventure despite the physical challenges she faced as her disease progressed. So the couple knew they wouldn't have to give up their travels once Virginia came under their care.

One cross-country road trip was especially memorable.

Virginia, whose sweet tooth rivaled a five-year-old's, loved candy. But not just for herself. Candy was the gift all her friends and family could count on for any occasion, great or small. So when the trio neared Abilene, Kansas, on a sunny summer day, it triggered a reminder that they would need to make their customary stop at the Russell Stover candy outlet.

Once inside the store, Virginia maneuvered a cart that served as both walker and candy treasure chest. Up one aisle and down the next, she loaded it up with boxes and boxes of her favorite sweet treats. Truffles, caramels, toffee bars. Hard candies, soft candies, peanut brittle. Dark chocolate, milk chocolate, crunchy chocolate. Surely something from each shelf was represented in Virginia's cart.

The three were having so much fun shopping for candies and chocolates that they forgot one little detail—until they walked out of the store.

It was 102 degrees. Even hotter in the car.

Oops.

"Okay, well, let's make sure to put this chocolate where it won't melt," said the practical Virginia.

But forget putting all that chocolate next to the air conditioning vents. It would be a miracle if they could fit it in at all—nearly every square inch of the car was already packed, and Virginia barely had enough space for herself in the back seat.

Ken looked again at the thermometer. Sure enough, still 102 degrees. As if his body didn't know it. Now used to working together like a smooth assembly line, Fran and Ken loaded the candy into every empty nook and cranny they could find inside the car. In between all the bags and Virginia's mobility paraphernalia—and in spaces they didn't even know existed—the couple squeezed countless boxes of Russell Stover's candies. An unparalleled feat to be sure.

While the chocolate came through unscathed, Ken and Fran did not. If people could melt, they did. They couldn't remember ever being so hot.

As they set out on the road again, quiet filled the car—until the crackling sounds began. With every little rustling of foil, lighthearted accusations flew back and forth as to just who might be sneaking a truffle or caramel from the boxes hidden among them.

And never for one minute did any of the three stop laughing. Not then and not as they crossed each city west of Russell Stover until they pulled into the driveway back home.

Cuttin' Loose

The Home Depot sign cast its orange hue on the parking lot like a rising sun spilling its warmth as Helenn and Joe pulled up. It had been just over a year since Joe had received the diagnosis of a rare neurodegenerative disease, and his active lifestyle was slowing down as he moved between walker and wheelchair. It helped Helenn to have such a spirited man for a husband, though; Joe was aware of what he could and couldn't control, and so he wasn't one to spin wheels over the way he wished his life could be. "We're all going to die from something," he would muse, "and PSP will be my something." Joe figured the journey would be a whole lot easier if he moved with his disease rather than resisted it.

He could also see the comedy in situations, and he wasn't about to give up his ability to laugh just because the disease sometimes put him in compromising situations.

Helenn had no choice but to adopt that attitude herself.

It was from this very frame of reference that the couple entered the Home Depot, Joe holding onto Helenn's arm as they walked. Their first stop would be the restroom; much to their relief, they had heard the Home Depot had a raised toilet. As Helenn was absorbing directions from the helpful greeter, Joe was quietly plotting his own adventure. Suddenly, he spied a motorized shopping cart sitting off in a corner, and his eyes lit up.

This was his chance to have some fun. He would be able to move. Fast.

Helenn turned back to tell Joe where they were going, but Joe was gone. *Oh gosh, this place is huge,* thought Helenn. *But at least I know he's in here somewhere.*

For the next half hour, Helenn peered up and down all the aisles. No Joe. She checked the restroom. No sign of him. She entered the paint section, rounded the kitchen remodeling area, then looked for him among the lamps. Back to front and side to side, she covered every square foot of concrete. Leaving the main home improvement building, she crossed over to the nursery. Plants and sod and hand-built gazebos stared her down, mocking her perplexity.

No matter where she went, Joe eluded her.

By now, Helenn was moving into frantic mode. Had he tipped over behind a row of heavy, rolled-up area rugs? Gotten trapped between kitchen counters? She quickly erased these scenarios from her mind; common sense told her he was safe, just creating a lark for himself, but for heaven's sake, where was this man of hers?

Flustered, Helenn approached the information desk.

"I'm looking for my husband," she blurted out. "He's riding on a motorized cart. I'm sure he's looking for me, too."

The clerk grinned. "Well, I haven't seen him. But we sure have been hearing about him."

Without another word to Helenn, the employee pulled out her walkie-talkie and made sure her crackling voice reached every other employee in the store: "The guy who's been cuttin' loose in the aisles, time to bring him in."

Joe and Helenn laughed all the way back to their car.

Dance Therapy

The adult day care center in town was a godsend. "Sure, I'm a barrel of laughs," quips JoAnn, "but Fred was used to a much larger social circle than just me. The adult day care center gave him an opportunity to be around people with similar challenges, so he didn't feel so alone. Getting out always sent him home with a stronger sense of wellbeing."

At least for the first year or so, before Fred's condition was too limiting, he was able to participate fully in the structured group activities the staff planned as a means of supporting participants' independence and personal growth. Three days a week, from 8 a.m. until 4 p.m., Fred felt welcome, safe, and understood. JoAnn noticed how her husband appeared physically, emotionally, and intellectually stimulated after taking part in enriching activities such as music, art, and day trips.

And dancing.

JoAnn would come early on dancing days and join her husband in a spin around the room, Ginger Rogers to his Fred Astaire. From the outside, onlookers saw a petite redhead staring up at her tall, blond man while three or four helpers assisted him in moving his legs. But between the two lovers, they had eyes only for each other. Astaire and Rogers' *Flying Down to Rio* had nothing on Fred and JoAnn gliding down the dance floor at the adult day care center. For those moments, all their cares whirred past like streaks of light from a glittering chandelier. No one was sick. No one was worried. Just two people bonded body and soul, swirling to the smooth cadence of songs from long ago, bathed in the sheer serenity of moving together to the rhythm of their life.

And then the music stopped. The helpers stepped into the background, and once again Fred was completely hers. She placed her hands into his balance belt, guided him to the door, and off they went to continue their life at home.

Recharged. Refreshed. Renewed.

Honestly, the Things a Caregiver Will Do

Germaine often surprised herself with how she reacted to the frequent shenanigans of her husband, Willie. In her mind, she thought she adhered quite admirably to her self-prescribed rules for being a loving caregiver. But every now and again, Willie would throw her for a loop, and she'd find herself doing whatever she needed to do to handle the situation.

The trip to the psychiatrist was one of those situations.

Germaine was hoping a psychiatrist could give her some insight into how Willie's mind operated. His antics were quite a conundrum. "Honestly," she had told his doctor, "why does the man do what he does?" When Willie's doctors were still plodding the confusing path of diagnosing such a rare disease as progressive supranuclear palsy, they had dismissed Alzheimer's disease, but did show concern about his struggles with strategizing and organizing.

Indeed.

Still fresh in Germaine's mind was the day she had come home with six new pairs of pants and shirts for him. She set the bag of goods in the closet. "Just leave them here, Willie. I'll help you try them on later," she said. An hour later, she checked in on him, and there he was in the bathroom, all his new clothes in a pile on the floor. She patiently picked them up and took them to his room.

Another hour passed, and Germaine felt uneasy about the silence. This time she found Willie in his closet, only by now he had pulled even more garments off their hangers and added them to his pile. She stoically hung each one back on its hanger and cautioned her husband to stop pulling them down.

Another hour passed. Remembering the inordinate amount of time he was able to devote to installing and removing batteries from all his flashlights, she feared the worst as she once again approached his room. Willie didn't fail to deliver. There he was, this time with just about every piece of clothing he owned, plus the new ones, piled high like a stack of fall leaves ready for a bonfire.

Enough of this patience stuff. Germaine exploded.

"If you take these down again, Willie, I'll kick you in the—" She didn't even finish her sentence, but it worked.

That's the kind of thing Germaine was dealing with on a regular basis.

One day, she had to make the trip with Willie to the closest major city to see his psychiatrist. She was hoping to gain some advice about how to deal with this increasing tomfoolery that Willie seemed powerless to control.

But driving into the city was not always clear sailing, and the evaluation itself would take a couple of hours. So before departing, Germaine took inventory of all the items Willie would need for the next several hours. *Walker? Check. Snacks? Check. Medication? Can't forget that.*

"Willie, here are your meds, but you won't need them till later. Now take care of them," she said kindly. She handed him the plastic pill baggie. *Let's see… jacket, sunglasses, a book for me to read.* She silently rattled off the mental checklist she had come up with specifically for outings with Willie.

"Okay, off we go."

As the couple got closer to their destination and downtown came into view, traffic thickened with cars pouring onto the freeway from every onramp. Suddenly, Willie shouted, "Turn around!"

"Wha-what?" Germaine was startled.

"I left my pills at home. Turn around."

Oh, goodness. What did he do with them? She pictured his bag of pills lying on the living room floor, or perhaps between the cushions of the couch. *So much for safekeeping.* She shrugged, and refocused her attention to the road.

Knowing Willie's psychiatrist held to a tight schedule, she didn't dare be late. She calmly explained to Willie that with traffic increasing, and with an hour's drive back to their house, they would never make their appointment on time if they tried to go back. But Willie refused her logic.

He launched into a tirade about his missing pills and wouldn't let go of it.

The cyclonic combination of Willie's ranting and the frenetic rush of cars was making her mind spin, and Germaine needed a minute to think. She looked to her right and made her way to the next exit as Willie continued his stubborn crusade. Off the freeway now, she pulled over to the curb and turned to face her husband. *How am I going to calm him down?* she wondered.

Then she had an idea. She reached into her purse and fumbled around. *Thank God,* she thought. *The Tylenol is still there.* She handed four tablets to Willie. They would be his placebos. "Well, look what I found. You didn't forget them after all. Take just two right now and save the other two for later."

Honestly, the things a caregiver will do, she rebuked herself, but only half-heartedly.

As she merged back onto the freeway and concentrated on negotiating traffic, Willie took advantage of her distraction to pop all four Tylenols.

During the evaluation Willie could barely stay awake, eventually nodding off altogether.

"What's going on here?" the doctor asked Germaine, motioning toward her slumbering husband.

"Well, it's like this . . ." Germaine spilled the whole story of the freeway drama.

The doctor listened and cringed. "So he didn't get his morning meds, and he did get four Tylenols. Well, I can't continue the evaluation today with Willie so sleepy. We'll have to reschedule."

As Germaine led her groggy husband to the door, the psychiatrist had one last question. "Why? Why did you give him Tylenol and not, say, gum or Life Savers?"

Germaine tossed all resolve to be the perfect caregiver out the window and spoke her mind.

"Sir, the man wanted his pills. At that particular moment, I would have given him anything he wanted just to keep him in the car and shut him up."

The doctor gulped.

Rising Above the "If Onlys"

Nestled in an outdoor playground far from frenzied city life, far from cell phone coverage, and best of all, far from daily reminders of their increasing limitations, the cozy cabin beckoned Ken and Audrey into its warm embrace. Breathtaking scenery, pristine air, and dramatic foliage served as a welcome sanctuary for the couple. Yes, the family cabin provided a perfect place for repose—or for staying busy. Both Ken and Audrey were of the latter bent.

But wherever they went, Audrey's illness followed. So during their frequent visits to the cabin, Ken would stay occupied with projects, while instructing Audrey not to get out of her chair unless he was there.

One day, while Ken was working on the deck, Audrey had sat empty-handed about as long as she could tolerate. She figured Ken must surely need her help by now. She'd just go check on him. She stood up and proceeded toward the kitchen where the bright window framed her husband, hard at work outside. She steadied herself as she walked along the walls until she came to the refrigerator. Ken had equipped the cabin with an RV refrigerator, which he'd placed inside a cabinet, unanchored to the ground. The rustic setup had served them well for many years.

Until this day.

Audrey had barely opened the refrigerator door when suddenly she felt something smack her with the speed and force of a wild turkey. Down she went, the weight of her oppressor bearing down on her crumpled body.

What Ken heard from outside was a loud thud. What he saw when he raced inside nearly stopped his heart. Audrey was trapped under the refrigerator—and cabinet—both of which had come crashing down on her. Without a second's delay, he hefted the bulky objects off his entrapped wife. All he saw was blood, bruises, and slashes. How she escaped any broken bones would forever be a mystery to him.

Ken's shock gave way to anger. If only she had listened to him. If only he had been inside when she approached the refrigerator. If only he didn't have to watch her constantly. If only their time at the cabin could be leisurely.

If only she weren't so sick.

When they got back to town, Ken sat down with his daughter, Gen, and told her the whole story. Overcome with terror and a sense of powerlessness, Gen gave up trying to hide her fears. "Dad, you're isolated out there at the cabin. You don't even have cell service. You yourself have suffered a brain injury. You can't keep taking Mom up there."

Ken fingered his white mustache as he listened to his daughter's fears. But he was tired of the if-onlys and what-ifs—they were almost more oppressive than the disease itself. Finally, he took off his glasses, set them on the table, and spoke his mind.

"Gen, we will absolutely continue to spend time at the cabin. We love it there." He shrugged. "If something happens, then something happens."

Ken picked up his glasses and looked longingly toward his wife.

"We can't stop living."

And they didn't.

Dealing with Delusions

When rheumatoid arthritis gripped Pam with a vengeance, she reluctantly turned her husband's physical care over to the staff at a nursing facility. She would now be able to look after herself better, something she had tried to do—but not sufficiently—when William needed her care around the clock. Once he was nestled safely in his room at the care center, Pam's role shifted to that of William's primary emotional support. But for the hard, physical work, at least, she was off the hook.

Or maybe not. All was not rosy in that little room of his, as it turned out, for delusions and hallucinations can be symptomatic of both multiple system atrophy and Lewy body disease.

The problem came in the form of a telephone. Because four of their five daughters lived out of state, the couple got permission to have a phone in William's room. That allowed him to stay in contact with his cherished girls, and Pam was consoled, too, knowing he could call her whenever he wanted.

This luxury, however, was short lived.

Apparently, William had made three phone calls to 911 reporting that his wife was missing. And he described her to a T. Pam was flattered that he remembered her so well, but the 911 operators were not amused. They knew where he was calling from and they reported him to the care center staff, whereupon William had to give up his phone. However, the facility did agree to an "Alzheimer's phone"—one that could receive calls but not dial out.

When presented with his replacement, an old-fashioned-looking thing, William didn't hide his disappointment and confusion. The former aeronautical engineer let everyone know that this phone simply wasn't going to cut it. He ran his hand over it. It had no buttons for heaven's sake.

He refused to use it.

But doggone it, he knew the buttons were in that room somewhere. Now Pam had a new job: taming William's delusions as he crawled around his room, combing the floor for those errant dial buttons.

So much for taking it easy.

Euphemisms and Threats

When a major tumble seriously injured Pat's husband, Bob, she immediately flew into "helicopter mode." Even though this had never been her style, she had to remind herself that her husband's safety was at stake, and that she had to save him from himself. With Bob's dignity first and foremost in her mind, she found ways to hover while silencing the conspicuous sound of her rotor blades.

"I'm not using any damn wheelchair," Bob grumbled, as the two got ready to make the daily trek to the neighborhood coffee shop.

No problem.

"This is your transport chair, Bob," Pat said, completely avoiding the word *wheelchair*. "And look, it has wheels; you can slide it into any table at the coffee shop. Lucky you." *Transport chair* worked for him.

The walker was equally disdained.

No problem.

"Let's grab your limo on our way out, Bob." He could embrace a *limo*.

Blue spots were an acceptable replacement for "handicapped parking," and *undies* disguised the indignity of wearing diapers.

But sometimes euphemisms didn't work, and Pat had to resort to threats. The guard belt was her biggest challenge.

Feeling like a lassoed steer, Bob was annoyed every time he felt Pat's firm tug on the guard belt around his waist when he tried to get in and out of the hot tub, walk up and down the stairs of their three-level house, or take a leisurely stroll. But Pat found a solution. She simply said it like it was. Without exactly threatening Bob, she led a *discussion* about how it would feel if his ribs were to break and blood were to splatter if he didn't wear the belt that prevented him from falling.

"Better to take the guard belt, Bob," was all she had to say.

Enough of those euphemisms.

Keeping Life Fascinating

R uth was suffering a deep interior crisis. "All my identity was gone once I became a caregiver," she reflects. "I went from being a professor to having no career to define me. I went from Jim's adventure partner to his caregiver. I was back in a town that I didn't know anymore, and no one knew me. The fascinating life Jim and I had created for ourselves was gone—and I was furious with the world."

And then, serendipity draped over her like the graceful branches of a willow tree, for when the student is ready, the teacher is there. A life-changing book fell into Ruth's hands, Dr. Henry Cloud and Dr. John Townsend's *How People Grow*. It transformed her worldview into one with profound meaning: she now saw herself as a woman who loves.

She realized that if she wanted to love her life, she needed to make sure it was interesting, stimulating, and enjoyable. And since Jim was her life, she had to start by keeping the fascination alive in *his* life. It was in her power to do so despite the trying circumstances of his illness, she believed. She wanted to be happy again for sure, and she wanted to give Jim the gift of a happy wife. He deserved that.

That very mission was the best way she could find to love her husband as herself.

To that end, Ruth sought out activities that Jim would enjoy, which included therapeutic horseback riding and attending retired firefighters' breakfasts. She invited old friends to come by and visit. She read the Bible to him, which helped him stay calm. They worked on crossword puzzles together, he providing the words, she scribbling them into the boxes.

She gave herself permission to put Jim before housework and to accept fatigue as a given, not a weakness.

She discovered the power of exercise. When Ruth recognized that she was gaining weight, she laughed it off at first. "Well, what can I say?" she says lightheartedly. "During his long meals—it took two hours on average—I had nothing better to do than engage in a little nibbling myself." But soon, the couple began an exercise regimen that worked for both of them.

Not only did hardy movement help her burn off those extra calories, but the endorphins improved her sense of wellbeing. It also improved her strength so she could lift Jim when needed. Even better, though, it strengthened Jim's legs. For an hour a day, faithfully, the two exercised side by side. Sitting poses. Leg lifts. Lunges. And sometimes a walk around the community center. They would use transfer poles to move along and a gait belt for balance.

She applied for a respite care scholarship from the county's Office on Aging, which paid for in-home caregivers so she could go out to lunch occasionally or attend her book club. Counseling and free caregiver support, also available to her from the county, helped her mission.

And she joined a support group. There, she found compassion, camaraderie, and understanding beyond anything she'd experienced to date. Just as important: she was able to garner the members' wisdom. Specifically, she learned that people actually travel with their patients. Fascinating. Maybe they would give it a try. Jim and Ruth had planned to go to Hawaii for their twentieth anniversary, so six months after learning of the demoralizing implication of Jim's illness, the couple thumbed their noses at the disease and took off for the Aloha State, power chair and transfer chair in tow, the wind at their backs.

"How did I do it?" Ruth asks. "I stopped being a victim. I learned to make my life fascinating by making Jim's life fascinating. We fed each other in that way."

Chocolate Cake Feast

Even in the throes of his debilitating disease, Fred showed his playfulness at every turn. On some days, his vacant look made him appear to be sleeping, even though his eyes were open. But JoAnn knew better. At any moment, her husband might break the silence with a sudden guffaw—her signal that he was rarin' to engage.

One evening, Fred's daughter, Sheryl, came to visit and brought with her a chocolate cake. She slipped it to JoAnn then sidled over to Fred, who was watching television. Dessert would come soon enough. For now, she wanted to have a little fun with her dad. To make sure he stayed as alert and active as he could, Sheryl had learned that playing catch with him did the trick. So she waved the cloth ball in front of him and motioned her intent to throw it to him. Propped up in his chair, Fred was poised to catch. And then he got ready to throw it back. But, tease that he was, he didn't want to make it too easy on his daughter. Putting on a helpless act, he dropped the ball so Sheryl would have to go get it. Then out came the burst of laughter, a subdued heh-heh, with a smile that bared his teeth. Sheryl loved that smile—but not when he was trying to get her goat.

Just then, JoAnn walked into the room. "Who wants cake?" she asked, looking directly at her husband.

The endearing smile Fred never lost during his illness spread across his face, followed by the hand signal that indicated yes, his wrist slightly bent as if knocking on a door. "You got it!" said Sheryl. Fred watched as his daughter seemed to take forever slicing through the thick, glistening frosting and three succulent layers of chocolate. He could hardly stand it as his wife tied the towel around him to keep his T-shirt and sweatpants clean. It took eons for JoAnn to find a cake-eating utensil. Finally—finally—Sheryl placed the cake in front of him, the feast he'd been waiting for. He was practically panting.

While Fred indulged in his treat, JoAnn and Sheryl were leaning over the island counter a few yards away, chatting. Ten or fifteen minutes passed before either woman noticed.

Silence.

Simultaneously their heads jerked toward Fred. There he sat, grinning, his face covered top to bottom in chocolate cake and frosting, like a one-year-old reveling in his first taste of sweetness. His hair. His ears. His forehead, mouth, and chin. Covered. Even his towel. Crumbs everywhere. Had any of it reached his mouth?

It didn't matter. The teasing in Fred's eyes told JoAnn and Sheryl they'd been had again.

JoAnn simply cut him another piece and let him have at it.

Chivalry Lost

One of Sonja's hardest trials was having to tell Ken he could no longer drive. It was a drastic step, but a terrifying experience left her with no choice.

The incident took place one day as they were getting ready to leave an event at a city park. Ken was ahead of her in his car. Suddenly, she let out a scream. She watched helplessly as Ken drove up onto the sidewalk—and straight into the park.

Sonja was shocked that her husband's driving skills had deteriorated so much. She had to put her foot down. Although the two hardly ever fought, Ken was fuming. "You're trying to control me," he insisted. "I just got confused for a minute, that's all."

Ken sulked and groused about it for the rest of the day, but Sonja didn't budge. The safety of a lot of people was at stake, after all, including his own. She understood why he was so angry—he was coming from a place of powerlessness and fear—but fury was not Ken's typical way of responding. He didn't even express sadness very often.

Except once.

That time involved his chivalry. It had always been Ken's way to open the car door for his wife, or to drop her off in front of a building during bad weather, then go park the car. Even while he was using a walker, he would still make it a point to open her door, wait till she got seated, then shuffle around to the other side of the car and do his best to wriggle his way into the driver's seat.

But his chivalry had to stop after Sonja took over the driving duties.

One evening, the couple went out together. Since their roles were now reversed, Sonja escorted Ken to his seat, buckled him in, then hoisted his walker into the trunk. Once settled in herself, she looked over at her husband. Tears were streaming down his face. A confusing whirlpool of compassion, tenderness, and sorrow churned in Sonja. She took his hand in hers and did her best to comfort him. But none of her reassurances could reach his heart.

With every word she spoke, his tears flowed anew.

Coffee Trials

Carol was something of a wise guy in her personal and professional life, so it surprised no one to find out that she was also a plucky patient. To be blunt, Carol's illness brought out her inner two-year-old: Stubborn. Cunning. But always with a twist of lovable mirth.

Like when she was drinking coffee.

Carol loved to indulge in her warm beverage—on her own terms. So each day, she'd accept the steaming cup, cradle it for a few minutes, then begin sipping.

While lying on her back.

It was the same story day after day. Her caretaker daughter, Andy, would notice that what had been a brilliant marigold Hanes T-shirt suddenly bore a slight coffee-bean hue. Time to help her mother change. Off with the stained shirt, on with the clean.

But then Carol would do it again. Her new, clean shirt drenched with coffee.

Time after time, Andy patiently reminded her mother to sit up while she drank her coffee. Time after time, Carol promised she would. And time after time, she leaned back before imbibing, as if lounging on a chaise, in perfect imitation of Cleopatra.

One day, after three changes of clothing, Andy had had it.

"Now, Mom, what should you do when you're drinking coffee?" Andy chided.

"Sit up," Carol uttered, a trace of mockery in her voice.

"Then why don't you?"

The words were slurred but resolute. "I can drink lying down."

An adult, parkinsonism version of *I can do it myself!*

That was Carol all right.

An Athlete and a Gentleman

In the early stages of his disease, Phil found himself having to balance his courteous nature with his athletic prowess—and occasionally having to juggle those with his expertise in furniture. One day, he walked into the office of a neurologist, a man whose interior design skills were on par with those of a sixth-grade camp counselor. The dark, wood-paneled walls closed in on the room, which was already filled to capacity with the only furniture he had: three stark, wooden chairs. Having been a furniture-store owner for many years, Phil could hardly hold back the flood of ideas for improvement he wanted to share. But he bit his tongue.

Instead, he focused on his task, which was to demonstrate his gait by walking across the room. Problem was, the room was so cramped that he couldn't take more than three steps, and how bad can a guy's gait be in three tiny steps? So, of course, he passed that test with flying colors.

Next, the neurologist tested Phil's strength by pushing down on his arms and legs, asking Phil to resist as best he could. Phil resisted—in spades.

Finally, the balance test. The doctor planned to come up from behind, push Phil, then catch his patient as he fell forward. In such a weakened state, most patients would fall forward.

But Phil was not most patients.

Still strong and athletic, he was ready when he felt the hand that was meant to topple him. He was ready when the neurologist heaved his weight at Phil, pushing on his muscular back.

And he was ready when the doctor flicked backward like a runner band, nearly face-planting into his wood-paneled wall.

Appointment over. I'm fine, Phil huffed to himself.

Fine indeed. At another appointment, in a different doctor's quarters, Phil had a chance to pepper his brawn with gallantry. The doctor was trying to explain the medical ramifications of her findings to Phil and his wife, Barb. But the couple were distracted by the precarious way she was perched on her chair; it was clearly falling apart, and they worried she would lose her balance and fall if they so much as exhaled. Finally, the doctor decided it was safer just to stand up while she talked. In unison, Phil and Barb breathed a sigh of relief, and could now concentrate on what the doctor had to say.

But Phil wasn't satisfied.

The doctor, open-mouthed, gasped when she saw her "impaired" patient bend down, pick up the chair, turn it over—and repair it right then and there.

An athlete and a gentleman. Yep.

Carolyn at the Bat

Phrases and entire verses shamelessly borrowed from
Ernest Lawrence Thayer's poem "Casey at the Bat."

The outlook wasn't brilliant when the bat got in the house.
Carolyn had been functioning on very little sleep—night after night
after night—as she tended to the nocturnal needs of her husband,
Dave. His trips to the bathroom, requests for water, even reminders to
make sure the phone was recharging in its cradle, were playing havoc
with her REM sleep. So she wasn't her most alert when Dave shouted,
"Carolyn! Quick! Something just flew in the window!"

Half asleep, she moaned, then straggled in near despair, clung to
that hope which springs eternal in the human breast that maybe . . . maybe
. . . she could go back to sleep.

No luck.

The dogs were howling, Dave was yowling. Something had to be
done. Ready to escort the pups outside, she flipped on the lights.

And shrieked.

A leather-colored bat came hurtling through the air, straight
toward her face. At first, Carolyn froze. Then she grabbed a baseball cap
and covered her hair so her nemesis wouldn't snarl its nasty body through
her strands.

"Bats don't get in your hair," Dave calmly advised. "That's
a myth."

"I don't believe you," she said, and threw on a sweatshirt for
additional armor.

She was now fully awake.

Carolyn looked over at her husband, then right back at the bat.
And again at her husband. Since Dave's eyesight and movement were

166

limited, there seemed but little chance of his getting to the bat.

She sighed a sigh and heaved a heave. Slowly reality crept in, then slammed her in the face: this was her fight to fight. With a deep breath, defiance flashed in Carolyn's eye, a sneer curled her lip.

Carolyn was at the bat.

Out of the bedroom she sprinted, banged the door behind her and headed to the kitchen where she snatched a broom and flashlight—then, unheeded, sped back to the bedroom. "Hold this!" she screamed as she threw the flashlight to Dave. Progressive supranuclear palsy had given Dave a grip of steel, so Carolyn rested assured that her husband would clutch that flashlight and not even know how to let go. While he shined the light on the bat, Carolyn stormed around the room pounding with cruel violence at the errant bat, the air shattered by the force of her blows.

Dave watched as her visage shone, her face grew stern, her muscles strained. He knew she wouldn't let that bat go by again. "Don't kill him! Open all the windows so he can go out," Dave hollered. *Darn animal lover,* snarled Carolyn in her mind. She yanked the curtains aside and pulled down the window, hoping to knock the bat out of the ballpark.

But gentle wasn't doing the trick. *Hmm,* Carolyn wondered, *what would a bat catcher do? Of course. Use a net.* So off she dashed to the garage for a fishing net. Dave, trapped in the bedroom with a crazed bat, continued to urge it to the window the only way he was able: by waving the flashlight wildly, a one-man fireworks show.

Carolyn returned, fishing net in hand, and climbed onto the bed where she cautiously lifted the net under the bat, who was resting momentarily on the ceiling directly above. While Dave aimed the flashlight on the net, Carolyn held her breath—and the bat flew right into her trap. Off the bed she hopped, strode to the window, emptied her quarry into the night air, and slammed those windows shut.

In this favored land of theirs, the moon was shining bright; no bands were playing anywhere, but here their hearts were light.

Carolyn high-fived her love and tumbled into bed. She wouldn't get enough sleep before the sun rose.

But she wouldn't have traded their adventure for anything.

Proper Church Wear

Virginia being Virginia, she never let a little life-threatening diagnosis get in her way of having fun, but it did change some of her long-held attitudes. For example, this proper lady had always thought it disgraceful for women to wear slacks to church. It showed a lack of respect, she asserted. She herself preferred that the clear, brilliant church windows cast their glow on her tasteful dress and Sunday best high-heeled shoes. It was her way of being reverential toward her God.

Those tiny heels were a concern to Virginia's daughter, Fran, however. Her mother was increasingly losing her balance, and it would take nothing to trip and break an ankle or a leg. Or worse, a hip. But Fran deferred to her mother as often as she could out of respect for her independence, and figured as long as she kept an eye on her, this was a small battle, best left unpicked.

One day after returning home from church, the family walked into the house from the garage, and Virginia proceeded directly to her downstairs apartment. This involved first walking up six steps, then around a corner and down a few steps, veering left down another small staircase, and finally descending the final flight of thirteen steps to her private dwelling. By then, Fran and Ken knew to watch their housemate closely, so they were ready and waiting, poised to lunge in case a thud should be lurking.

Suddenly one of Virginia's shoes fell off. Without a second's hesitation, Ken was there to catch her just in the nick of time.

"Now can we stop wearing those little heels?" said Fran. Obediently, Virginia slid right over to the closet and tossed her shoes inside, where they would stay forevermore.

Flat, comfortable shoes would be just fine for church.

And following, not far behind, were slacks.

Man Cave

One thing Willie refused to relinquish, given his new life of successive surrenders, was his coveted garage. No way. It was his sanctuary, his creative den, the place where he could live as a PSP patient without anyone watching.

But in her unobtrusive way, Germaine was always watching. She had to, because Willie didn't know his own strength. And for a period of time, she had to be extra vigilant, because Willie had a habit of tossing everything into the garbage. Everything. One time it was his glasses, another time, his teeth. Usually they were less valuable items, but still, Germaine had long ago learned to check the trash cans around the house regularly.

One day, after she had purchased a large supply of batteries, Germaine noticed they were missing. "Oh, that Willie," she muttered. She went immediately to the kitchen receptacle, his usual dumping ground. No batteries. She went to each part of the house, dug through the garbage, and room by room came up empty handed. "Now this is confusing. Where are those batteries?"

Then the idea came to her like a swarm of fireflies on a summer night: the garage. Minutes later, she was at the door to Willie's "man cave," and sure enough, there was her husband, with batteries spread all over his workbench as he tried different pairs of them in each of the six new flashlights he had bought on his last visit to the store.

Changing batteries to see if they would work had become a favorite pastime that kept him entertained for hours. Watching Willie unwrap and sort those batteries hour after hour was reminiscent of the glee she saw in her children when they would bang on pots and pans— albeit while leaving their expensive toys to gather dust in their rooms.

But with a certain sense of relief, Germaine embraced Willie's workspace. She saw it as a different kind of caregiver, one that offered her respite from the mischief he seemed to generate inside their home: his bumping into furniture, snits when he wasn't satisfied, projects he created that never quite seemed to come together. The garage was small, clean, and free of hazards. Safe. And he was happy in there. What could possibly go wrong?

One balmy afternoon as the sun took its four o'clock position in the sky, Germaine's intuition tapped her on the shoulder. Time to go check on Willie, it prodded. She approached the garage and quietly opened the door.

"Oh my gosh, Willie!" she shrieked, clutching her heart.

There stood her husband, perched atop a fourteen-foot ladder.

"You get down from there right now." She steadied the ladder and beckoned him to start climbing down. "What in the world were you doing up there?"

"Oh, just seeing what's in the rafters," he said, wobbling on each and every rung.

Once safely on the ground, Willie wiped his hands on his shirt. "Little dusty up there," he said casually as he sat down again to rearrange his flashlights.

Drive-Thru Service

It was a sunny day, but not warm enough to spend much time outdoors. On days like this, when Joe simply needed a change of scenery, his wife, Helenn, would take him to the supermarket, where she could push him a few times around the inside of the store in a great big loop. So off they went to shop for groceries.

They followed their routine. Helenn sat Joe in his wheelchair, rolled him from the house to the car, lifted him out of the chair and guided him into the seat, buckled him in, then folded the chair and stuffed it into the trunk. When they got to the store, they reversed the process. Quite a team, Joe and Helenn.

After their supermarket tour, Joe told Helenn he'd like to shake things up a bit and sit in the back seat for the trip home. *Why not?* Helenn unlocked the car door, pushed Joe's wheelchair right up to it, maneuvered him into the back seat, and closed the door. Then she slid her plastic grocery bags onto her wrists, pushed the wheelchair around to the back of the car, opened the trunk, folded the chair, placed the chair in the trunk and her bags on the chair, and closed the trunk. *There,* she congratulated herself. *You're good.*

Helenn secured her seatbelt and peered into the rearview mirror. Cautiously, she backed out of her space, then turned the steering wheel and drove forward.

"Whoa!' she screamed, slamming on the brakes. Without warning, a small child had darted out in front of her.

Helenn exhaled her relief. Catastrophe averted. But unbeknownst to her, another catastrophe was unfolding in the back seat.

It started with the familiar thud.

"Joe, are you okay?" she asked, only mild panic filling her voice. No sound.

Helenn turned around just long enough to see Joe, not in his seat where she'd personally placed him moments ago, but on the floor, wedged between the front and back seats. Almost completely sideways. And stuck. Really stuck. She pulled into an empty parking space and set about trying to dislodge him.

No luck.

Helenn got back into the car and plopped herself down on her seat to consider her options. *Hmm. I could flag someone down to help me,* she thought. She looked around and saw only a frail, gray-haired senior and a young mother with an infant in her arms and toddler in tow. She thought about running back inside and asking an employee for help. But when she took another peek down at her scrunched-up husband, hopelessly sandwiched between the seats, she decided she'd better not leave him alone.

Then her eyes caught a familiar sight just down the street: a fire station. "Can you hang on, Joe? I know what to do," she said over her shoulder.

Off to the fire station headed Helenn and Joe.

It wasn't immediately obvious where a person should park to visit the paramedics, but Helenn pulled off to the side of the station and turned off the ignition. The garage facing the busy street housed the same red-and-white ambulances that showed up frequently at Joe and Helenn's home.

There was no welcome mat beckoning her inside, so Helenn crept around the back, where she found a door. Two firemen answered her knock.

"Excuse me," said Helenn. "My husband has PSP, and—"

She stopped as their eyes glazed over. She needed to make this simple.

"Progressive supranuclear palsy. It's like ALS."

Blank stares.

"Lou Gehrig's disease."

Nods of recognition.

"Anyway, he's stuck between the front and back seats of the car and I can't pry him out. And his limbs are too stiff for him to help me."

The firemen rose to the occasion. From out of nowhere bounded four more strapping men who followed Helenn to the car—biceps bulging, six-pack abs making their presence known. As if their rescue tactics had been designed for this exact scenario, the team took their posts. Two of the guys extricated Joe's feet, two worked on his head, a fifth supported his middle, while a sixth orchestrated the entire effort. Like a crane at an excavation site, the human machine lifted Joe out from between the seats. Then the six men hoisted him above their shoulders and carried him in a supine position like a victorious sports team parading their hero before his fans.

After they strapped Joe into the front seat, they offered to drive the couple home.

"Oh, that won't be necessary," said Helenn. "My mistake was not remembering to belt him in. I was so distracted back at the store. But we'll be fine now."

Before she drove off, she rolled down the window.

"Thank you all so much. I suppose you're often called on to help," she said.

The nearest paramedic chuckled.

"Well, yeah, but I can definitely say we've never provided drive-thru service before."

Clicker Capers

F red had absolute jurisdiction over the television remote control. This served several purposes. First and foremost, it gave him independence while he was losing his freedoms right and left. But it also satisfied his need for repetitive motion, and fed his fascination with cause and effect. And then there was the advantage for JoAnn: she didn't need to be with him every time he wanted to change the channel. In fact, she didn't pay much attention at all to what her husband watched on TV—that was her time to get things done around the house.

One day something strange showed up in the hands of the UPS delivery man. "Fred?" asked JoAnn. "Why did the UPS man just deliver a vacuum?"

"Oh, I ordered it from the TV," he communicated. "Did the year's supply of bags come too? And the extra attachments?" JoAnn groaned. *Of course,* she grunted to herself. *The but-wait-there's-more! bonuses.*

The next surprise was the sudden appearance of an internet connection, which JoAnn had no idea what to do with. Yep. Fred had fingered in that order on his clicker, too.

But the most unsettling was when the teenaged boy who occasionally sat with Fred while JoAnn went out pulled her aside and whispered, "I can't watch TV with Fred. I don't want to see that stuff."

JoAnn finally learned what "that stuff" was when Fred's son came over hoping to watch the football game. His eyes bugged out. What he saw on the screen was completely out of character for his father. Fred was not watching football.

It took two hours to cancel Fred's latest purchase: a three-month subscription to a porn channel. But wait! If he ordered immediately, he would get an extra month free. And indeed he had.

In Your Face, PSP

Ken and Audrey took to traveling like hobos to a train. Six treks to Europe and Asia—all planned in detail by Audrey—as well as trailer trips from shore to shore in the U.S. became the couple's hallmark. Even when PSP threatened to curtail their journeys, the two of them managed to keep the monster at bay and continue on their merry way.

A brief episode on one of their trips, while the two were still in blissful ignorance of Audrey's condition, disturbed Ken. Audrey was at the wheel when suddenly she stopped and pulled over. "Ken . . . I . . . I can't drive," she said. She hesitated before turning toward him. "I can't see." At the time, neither had any idea this vision problem was a symptom of a degenerative neurological disease that would turn their lives upside down; they simply switched seats, and Ken drove the rest of the way.

Later, after a three-week road trip with Audrey's sister and brother-in-law, a letter arrived for Ken. It was from Audrey's sister. "Something's wrong with Audrey," she wrote. She went on to cite her observations that Audrey hadn't talked much on the trip and that she was much more passive than usual, not the take-charge woman they'd always known. She'd noticed, too, that Audrey's eyes were irritated from not blinking.

Ken's reaction was a combination of hurt and anger. *I've been with Audrey for a long, long time; don't tell me what to think*, he huffed to himself.

But his sister-in-law's comment bothered him more than he wanted to admit. With time, all of Audrey's symptoms converged into an official diagnosis of progressive supranuclear palsy, which clamored for recognition as the tyrant it was. Ken wondered if he was pushing Audrey too far. Questions hovered over him like mosquitoes at an otherwise pleasant campsite. Should they stick closer to home? Should they sell the trailer? Were they going to let illness win?

Ken and Audrey sold their travel trailer.

But then, as if to thumb their noses at that horrid disease, they bought another trailer—and put 4,500 miles on it that very year. Take that, PSP.

Taking Turns

Pam and her husband, William, found plenty of opportunities to see the funny side of their life together, and funny was often tender at the same time.

One week, Pam was awake four nights in a row because of William's constant stumbling and falling while trying to get to the bathroom. He couldn't abide being wet in or near his bed, which happened frequently despite his Depends. So he was up and down and back and forth, several times each night.

Between his bathroom visits, stumbles, and occasional thuds, Pam was awake for four straight nights as she attended her husband's needs.

On the last of these vigils, while camped on the couch outside the bedroom door, she tried to get up to use the bathroom herself. But she couldn't. Almost paralyzed from the pain of her own rheumatoid arthritis, she had to roll off the couch and crawl across the floor to get herself there.

When the sun finally rose, casting its hopeful rays on their home, Pam was enshrouded in the shade of total exhaustion. She shuffled into the bedroom where William was sleeping. Seeking closeness, she slipped in next to him, not planning to wake him.

But when his eyes opened, she couldn't help herself. "Can I take a turn napping while *you* watch *me* sleep?" she joked.

She doesn't remember falling asleep, but she does remember what she saw when she woke out of a deep slumber: there was William lying next to her, his head resting on his hand, staring at his beauty as she slept.

What revitalized Pam even more than the luxurious nap was William's love and caring as he watched his wife get some much-needed rest.

And the Oscar for Best Supporting Actress . . .

As Bob's health declined, Pat's acting skills sharpened. Firmly in the clutches of the impulsive behavior that is symptomatic of his disease, Pat's husband would spend hours punching the buttons on his insulin pump and endlessly clicking the universal TV remote. Pat had to do something to break his habit. But like anyone else with his condition, Bob had a nearly superhuman grip, and no matter what bodybuilding position Pat assumed, she simply could not wrest those objects from his hands.

So she did what so many of her fellow caregivers did: she took the batteries out of the remote control and handed the useless device back to him, which he happily played with—for two days.

But while Bob's neurological disease wreaked havoc on his body, his vibrant mind was still there. He was no fool. When he saw the lack of cause and effect between his button punching and the picture on the screen, he let Pat know he was onto her ruse: "You took the batteries out of the remote. Give me one that works!"

Well, nice try, she thought. *I wish he would show as much interest in the bells as he does in that darn remote.* Pat had placed miniature bells in the areas where Bob sat so he could alert her if he needed anything. But most of the time, Bob eschewed the bells and just stood up to go help himself— or worse, tried to make his way up the stairs without assistance.

But Pat held her tongue. Her guiding principle in being Bob's caretaker was always this: be with him where he is.

One morning, "where he was" required her best acting.

Bob was in a flustered state.

"I need my pen," he mumbled. "It got stuck between the mattress and the headboard, and I can't reach it." He continued with talk of a report he needed to finish, one which Pat recognized as an environmental report he had already written—five decades earlier.

He had been stuck in another one of his dreams.

Later, a similar problem.

"Where's the key?" he asked.

Since Bob didn't drive, Pat was confused. "Which one are you looking for?"

"That big, flat one. It's gotta be around here someplace." Bob looked determined. As soon as he described the key, Pat knew what he was talking about. The missing "big, flat key" unlocked their house in another part of the country, where they had lived forty years prior.

"I've got time to help you find it tomorrow, and I promise I will," Pat said, knowing he was trapped in another dream. "Now let's go get our coffee."

But Bob's mind didn't let go of the dreams. An hour later, the same question lingered. "Where is that key?"

True to her guiding principle, Pat stayed with Bob in the moment, knowing the key was real for him. She gave her best, Oscar-worthy performance yet by dramatically sweeping through the nearby rooms, then returning to report that the key was probably right in front of them, but it just didn't want to be found.

Bob bought it.

Ticket to Freedom

It was time to get rid of the exasperating lemon that was their Chevy Tahoe. Ruth and her husband, Jim, had owned it for years, but now that Ruth was the only one driving, she didn't want it anymore. Period. End of discussion.

"No!" said Jim, continuing the discussion. The Tahoe fit the image he desired—powerful, tough, manly—and he was not ready to relinquish it, not on top of everything else his disease had stolen from him.

But the last straw for Ruth came the day she left Jim alone for a few minutes to run to the post office. As she got into the truck to drive home, the engine refused to turn over—yet again. *Great,* she thought. *Just what I need when Jim is home alone.* She tried calling him several times, but he wasn't answering his cell phone. So she waited for a tow truck. Waited for the mechanic's estimate. Waited for a ride to the rental car facility. By the time she drove up to their house, several hours later, she feared the worst. Sure enough, when she opened the door, there was Jim, sprawled on the floor, having fallen out of his wheelchair. His cell phone had tumbled out of reach. "No more!" she declared in that moment.

As had been her lifelong pattern—and even more so since becoming her husband's caregiver—Ruth seemed to attract serendipity like lavender does butterflies. So she hoped for the best when she walked into the car dealership the next day. As it turned out, she had chanced upon an enterprise with a heart. After the salesman heard Ruth's story, he knew exactly how to help the couple: not only did Ruth and Jim get all their money back under the "lemon law," but they were able to buy, at cost, a minivan outfitted with a wheelchair lift. This now gave the couple all the accouterments they needed. No more worries about stalled engines. Lots of room for Jim's equipment and supplies. A way to quench their wanderlust. It was their ticket to freedom.

Not that Jim appreciated the image this van projected. But knowing he would do anything for her, Ruth easily brought him on board. "It's not for you, Jim. It's for me."

Period. End of discussion.

The Doorbell

By the time Fred was in the throes of his neurodegenerative disease, and his wife, JoAnn, fully into the routine of caring for him, the two had spent over thirty years developing the lighthearted, teasing relationship that defined their marriage. Even when Fred could no longer articulate his witty banter, he communicated playfulness with his eyes. Later, when his words were slurred, his voice only a whisper, he still found ways to engage with those he loved.

Beneath his increasingly frail exterior was a mind of steel, but sometimes Fred's lack of impulse control caused JoAnn's heart to stop. Case in point: When Fred needed something, he would simply get up out of his chair, forgetting that he was no longer able to walk. More than once JoAnn had sought muscle power from neighbors to lift her husband off the floor. Unfortunately, in their three-story house, JoAnn couldn't always hear Fred: he was in one room, but she had phone calls to return in another, beds to make upstairs, and laundry in the basement. No, this wasn't going to work. She'd have to find a way for Fred to summon her when he needed. JoAnn tapped into her creativity and came up with the perfect solution.

A portable doorbell.

All Fred had to do was punch the button. And since JoAnn would have the receiver with her wherever she went, she could be at Fred's side within seconds.

Of course, Fred and JoAnn had to have a little fun with this new arrangement. So did Fred's daughter, Sheryl, who visited often. A chip off the old block, Sheryl helped create their comical scenario: She referred to her father as "Fred with his two servant girls." JoAnn and Sheryl would be there when he dropped the remote, when he needed a glass of water, when the glare through the patio door was too much.

When he simply missed their company.

The most entertaining thing about the doorbell was that it came with twenty-five musical scores, and JoAnn and Sheryl got their jollies from changing up the songs. Fred never knew which tune would blare when he beckoned his servants—and he couldn't wait to see which personas they would assume.

They could be hams, those two women.

The *Lone Ranger* song, known to music aficionados as Rossini's *William Tell Overture*, might sound like this: "I'm on my way, Ke-mo-sah-bee!" Sheryl might wave her arms as if twirling a lariat, then stop at her dad's feet and look puzzled. "Who's this masked man, anyway?"

Beethoven's Ninth Symphony, the *Ode to Joy*: JoAnn might bow like a symphony conductor. "Ludwig at your service, my dear. I almost didn't hear you. I may be going deaf."

"Santa Claus is Coming to Town": JoAnn might pop her head around the corner. "Better not pout."

Well, these scenarios may or may not have been quite as Tony award-worthy as described, but the result was the same every time the two caregivers responded to Fred's call.

He smiled.

And smiled.

And smiled.

He seemed never to tire of their antics. He was having too much fun. In fact, JoAnn's pretty sure she saw him drop the remote a time or two.

On purpose.

Dancing Love Letters

Sonja and her husband, Ken, gradually redefined their lifestyle as his condition deteriorated. But what might have felt like a loss actually offered them gifts, for in their new, simpler existence, they discovered exultation in the ordinary. Ants, formerly pests, fascinated them with their strength. The miracle of flowers sprouting took on more profound meaning for them. When birds made their appearance outside, the two took notice as they never had before.

And in their simplicity, intimacy and tenderness blossomed in ever new ways.

One evening, the two were settled in their leather easy chairs watching TV when a Pat Boone infomercial came up. Soon, strains of the song "Love Letters in the Sand" filled the room, and Ken couldn't resist.

"Shall we dance?" he asked.

For the next few minutes, the pulse of the love song guided the rhythm of their movements:

> *On a day like today*
> *We pass the time away*
> *Writing love letters in the sand.*

The lyrics washed over them with deeper levels of meaning:

> *You made a vow that you would ever be true.*
> *Now my broken heart aches*
> *With every wave that breaks*
> *Over love letters in the sand.*

For those few minutes, the two danced their love story. Ken

simply stood and swayed, embraced by the love of his life.

That night was the last time the couple ever danced together.

31 Choices

After a long day of caring for Mike by herself, Annette was relieved to have help in the evening, as her vitality was waning by then. "It's amazing how much energy it takes to give Mike choices," she says. "One of the biggest heartaches was to watch his options dwindle. He was always such an independent man; that had to be a killer for him." Indeed, Annette had made a promise to herself that Mike's dignity would be the underpinning for every decision she made.

Which is why she was thrilled when the home health care agency sent The Patient One—capitalized, like God—to care for Mike. Every evening, this compassionate, sensitive woman, who shared Annette's commitment to Mike's self-respect, would prepare his favorite dessert: ice cream. Her nightly ritual was the same each time. From the freezer, she'd pull out as close to thirty-one flavors as she could, which was usually about a half dozen by the time her arms were full. One by one, she'd present them to Mike for his approval. She'd read the labels and hold a one-way conversation with him about the benefits of each.

"Chocolate marble fudge tonight, Mike?" she'd begin, holding the picture on the carton at his eye level so he could see it. "Now, this one has 130 calories per half cup, and it's made with real cream."

No response.

"What about Italian ice? Would you like to try a sample?"

Again, no response.

"What would you say if I offered you bubble gum ice cream? Just kidding. It's got actual gumballs in it—you're not getting that."

And so it went. One by one she carried them back to the freezer as Mike narrowed his choices, and sometimes back out again for him to reconsider.

And just when she thought he had made his final decision, the

186

process would start all over again.

By the time Mike dug into his evening treat, his bowl would be filled with four different scoops, four balls of varying colors and flavors to tickle his palate.

All his choice.

Escape Artist

Barb and her husband, Phil, kept up their date nights, even well into his illness. The only adjustment they had to make was when Barb became the chauffeur as Phil's peripheral vision declined.

On a particularly romantic evening, a slice of the moon forming a grin and stars splashed across the night sky, the couple drove to the movie theater. Phil's condition was progressing so slowly they sometimes hardly noticed the changes, but that night he discovered his latest limitation: he couldn't get out of Barb's low-to-the-ground convertible.

Barb noticed.

Without a second thought, she jumped out of her seat and ran to the other side to help.

She pulled.

She tugged.

She grunted and groaned.

But Phil would not budge. He simply couldn't muster the coordination he needed to duck under the roof and get out.

So Barb got creative.

The lifelong-athlete-now-apparently-turned-escape-artist flipped back the convertible top, stood up in the car, and, balancing her husband, turned him around, got one leg out, then went back to extricate the other.

There.

With Phil freed at last, the two of them sauntered into the theater as if they owned the world.

Two Bucks

Callae and her daughter Deri watched the scene with amusement. Even in the grips of his illness, their husband and father, Lee, was savoring his family.

"Grandpa Beaver, I cleaned up all the apples in the yard," said Deri's young son, Zach, using the family's term of endearment for him.

"Well, maybe you need a little walkin' around money, then," suggested Lee. And with that, Zach sauntered out of the room proudly jingling the coins in his pocket.

A few minutes later, he returned. "Grandpa Beaver, how much would you pay me to pick up all the doggy poops in the yard?"

Lee grunted, doing his best to project the image of a cheapskate. He had always tried to do the same with his daughter, so Deri knew what would come next. Zach stood waiting for his grandpa's go-ahead to start scooping for pay. "So how much, Grandpa?"

"Oh . . . I think . . . maybe . . . two bucks," said Lee, then chuckled as he watched his grandson scamper out the door to earn his fortune.

Callae glanced at the pictures on the mantel. In one, Zach and Lee were lying on their backs, heads resting on their hands, the triangles of their folded arms jutting out to their sides—male bonding at its finest. Next to it was a black-and-white photo of a young Deri, in a nearly identical pose a generation earlier, the two catching a few winks after one of Lee's graveyard shifts.

Lee adored his little girl. His plan had been to have six daughters, each named Shelley, but instead he channeled all the playfulness he would've given those six into his only child.

Clearly, Deri had her father's heart.

Father and daughter had an ongoing joke that wove itself throughout Lee's illness like ribbons on a maypole. Somewhere along the line, Deri had developed an obsession with bears. In fact, Lee often called her "Dooza Bear." So when she first caught a glimpse of the exquisite jewels of The Golden Bear, a pricey jewelry store in Vail, Colorado, she became enamored of their products. She made a habit of leaving dog-eared catalogs in Beaver's view, just in case he was looking for a gift for the one he called his favorite, albeit only, daughter.

Lee's quip was the same each time: "Sure, I'll give you two bucks." *Lotta good that'll do*, Deri always thought. And her dad knew it; his smile betrayed him.

When Lee died, his desire to take care of the ones he loved lived on. Two days before he passed away, he had signaled to Callae that he had something important to ask. In halting whispers he managed to say, "Papa Bear . . . charm . . . Deri . . . birthday. Will you?" Callae did exactly that.

And so it was that on Deri's birthday two months later, she opened the gift box and found a silver Papa Bear charm bracelet with a note from her father. "You'll always be my little girl," it said.

Deri has never removed her bracelet, her only visible connection to her dad.

As for Callae, every time she sees that Papa Bear charm bracelet on her daughter's wrist, she's reminded of the amazing man who brought so much richness to the life of his family.

Far more than two bucks' worth, that's for sure.

Wedding Vows

It took a lot of effort for Dave to communicate the desire that burned within, but Carolyn listened until she had it straight.

"Let's go to Loveland and renew our wedding vows," he said in halting phrases. He'd done his research the year before. The Loveland Ski Area in Colorado, just an hour from their home, held group "Mountaintop Matrimony" ceremonies—on Valentine's Day, of course, to befit its name. It was November, and their anniversary was coming up soon, but he really wanted to do it up big this year. Even though Valentine's Day was almost three months away, he needed Carolyn to make the reservation. His imagination was frothing with anticipation of the beauty they would witness. He and the love of his life, bundled in weatherproof wedding gear—whatever that would look like—the cold mountain air whipping their faces under the sapphire skies of the Rocky Mountains.

The previous year, he'd not been so lucky. He'd left a message with the outfit at Loveland that he wanted to surprise his wife with an anniversary she'd never forget: renewing their wedding vows on top of the world. But he never got a call back. He knew his speech was slurred. *Darn disease.* Had they thought he was drunk, like so many others did? Is that why they'd ignored his request? Well, this year his condition had declined considerably, so he knew he'd better enlist Carolyn's help.

Carolyn didn't know any of this had happened. So she was taken aback by his suggestion. "Loveland? You mean the ski slope? Wedding?" she asked. She couldn't imagine where they would hold such a fete. She strained her ears to understand the mumblings that harbored Dave's excited plans.

"Yes. It's their annual 'Marry Me and Ski for Free Mountaintop Matrimony,'" explained Dave, animation trying to break through his flat affect.

"Mountaintop," Carolyn repeated cautiously.

"Yeah, twelve o'clock sharp outside the Ptarmigan Roost Cabin. It's at an elevation of 12,050 feet." Carolyn was a pro at sensing his enthusiasm even if an outsider couldn't see it on his face. And he was showing a little bit too much zeal for her comfort.

"12,000 feet up?" Carolyn was getting nervous. "How do we get up there?"

"Chairlift." Dave cast his "duh" look. "Takes only twelve minutes to get to the top."

Carolyn relaxed. She could probably figure out how to get him on and off the chairlift with a little help from the staff. After all, they'd gone zip lining in the Philippines while he was sick, and lived to tell about it. *This might be interesting. And it's obviously important to Dave,* she thought. Her mind traveled back to their twenty-fifth anniversary—in Australia. She smiled. It touched her that Dave would still plan exotic anniversaries for them, as exotic as they could be given his physical condition. *We'll do this,* she decided.

"Well, if the lift will bring us up and down the mountain, that sounds doable," she said.

Dave shifted uncomfortably, then grunted.

"What," said Carolyn. The big "but" was coming. She just knew it.

"But the rules are that we have to ski or snowboard down after the ceremony. No chairlifts for the return trip."

Carolyn gulped. Dave was close to death. His deterioration over the last few months had been rapid. He seemed to know his life was coming to an end, so how did he think he could ski down a mountain?

"Dave." She embraced him. "Let's plan something that doesn't involve schussing down a mountain. Let's renew our wedding vows right here! We'll ask Bill to officiate," she said, referring to Dave's longtime close friend, a minister. "We can still do it for Valentine's."

Dave nodded reluctantly. Of course he knew better, but Dave wouldn't be Dave if he didn't dream big.

"Now don't you dare die on me before Valentine's Day," Carolyn teased. But she wasn't really kidding.

When their anniversary rolled around on November 19, Dave

presented Carolyn with a gift. She raised her eyebrows. *He can barely move. How could he have gotten me a present?*

She fingered the box. "Blanca took me to the jewelry store," he said. He explained how even though he couldn't see, his daytime caretaker had made his wishes known to the salesperson: he wanted to add a charm to Carolyn's Pandora bracelet, already laden with mementos of special times together. It was his tradition.

Carolyn slowly opened the box and lifted the charm from its cotton bed. Engraved on the jewel was a number: 32.

Thirty-two years a couple. Life partners. In that moment, the joy she felt silenced the fears she had been trying to keep at bay.

Thanksgiving and Christmas came and went, and Dave glided through them despite the specter of death hovering over him. Keeping her eyes on February 14, Carolyn couldn't imagine how Dave could hang on that long given how weak he was. She called Bill and moved the renewal-of-vows ceremony to January 28, as close to Valentine's Day as she dared risk.

Dave surprised Carolyn in two ways. First, on the big day, he presented her with flowers, chocolates, and a card at their private ceremony. And second, he not only lived until Valentine's Day, he stayed with her for thirteen days after that.

Carolyn grinned in gratitude. Once again, Dave had planned an exquisite anniversary celebration.

Their last.

Ace

Del and June's boating friends had come up with a bright idea for a party: a golf tournament. No, not of the caliber June used to take part in when she was an avid golfer. Those days were gone. But she could handle the putting contest, she thought.

Better than that, she intended to win.

Bring it on!

Del had learned long ago there wasn't much that could hold his wife back.

So on the day of the tournament, he helped her into the golf cart, and across the fairway they rode, the sun glinting off the narrow metal head of her putter.

When they stopped, Del helped June out of the golf cart with the finesse of a personal trainer, and assisted her in walking up to the green. He fully expected that she would fall at some point, but he knew not to hover over his wife when she was in "resolute mode." He handed her the putter and let her have at it, then walked to the sideline to listen for the thud.

It never came.

Del watched as June put her best techniques into play. Keeping her eyes over the ball, posture and stance shifting as her balance allowed, and doing her best to keep her shoulders level, she picked her entry point and swung her club.

Del turned away after that. He admired her form—and he would tell her so afterward—but he wasn't sure she was going to have much success in this tournament. It would break his heart to see that look of disappointment on her face.

The time seemed to drag and then suddenly, the sound of cheering. Del turned to look, and what he saw forced a loud "Yes!" from his mouth.

There was June, waving her club, triumphant over winning the golf match.

Packed to the Gills

Despite relatively minor inconveniences, Fran and her husband, Ken, laughed their way across the United States with Fran's mother, Virginia, on road trips that defied Virginia's deteriorating condition.

By now, the two caregivers knew exactly how to pack for a trip. After an unfortunate incident one year when there was barely enough room in the car for both Virginia *and* her dozens of candy boxes from the Russell Stover outlet store, the trio purchased a van for future trips.

And they managed to fill that to the brim, too.

Picture this: A Toyota van is parked in front of a motel, ready to begin day two of a three-day, two-night road trip. Fran helps her mother step onto the footstool, then watches her grab the handgrips inside and swing herself onto the seat that has been cleverly covered with polyester so Virginia can slide easily across it. With the doors closed and everyone's seatbelt fastened, Ken now heads out of the parking lot.

Every inch of space in the van—from front to back, side to side, and floor to ceiling—is crammed with every accessory that will make Virginia's life on the road easier: walker, potty chair with handles to place over toilet seats in the motels, shower stool, tray with runners to slide under her chair so she can get closer to tables, oxygen concentrator, suitcases, coolers, and boxes of food. Ken and Fran had packed all this equipment before they set out from home, then they took it out and set it all up in the motel room last night, repacked it this morning, and will unpack it again tonight. They'll repeat the entire process on the return trip.

Everything that belongs to Virginia is inside the van.

Packed. To the gills.

No one can even see the five-foot, two-inch, bespeckled

octogenarian in this scene. No one can express amazement at how wrinkle-free her skin is, how still-brown her hair is, how lively her spirit.

All a person can see, as the trio drive off, is a small hand belonging to Virginia waving out the window.

Putting Out the Flames

"Let's go shopping," suggested Germaine. Browsing the aisles was therapy for her and her husband, Willie. For one thing, Germaine wouldn't have to worry about Willie's frequent falling, like she did at home when he shunned his wheelchair in favor of gripping the walls as he walked, or pushing his wheelchair ahead of him so fast that he would pull it back on himself, causing a bad fall. The popular, big-box stores were all set up for someone who was disabled, as long as he was safely confined in his electric wheelchair. This would actually be a time when Germaine could unwind a little.

The automatic doors parted as the couple entered the store, the bright aisles of everything-you-could-ever-possibly-want shamelessly flirting with them. Germaine had barely finished scanning the strategically placed impulse-buy rack when she sensed an absence next to her. Willie was gone.

Crash! Thud.

The commotion had come from several aisles over, but this time Germaine didn't rush to the scene. She already knew what had happened. Willie had torn off through the aisles like a feral rodent escaping its predator, and had knocked down a display. She could even predict what would happen next: he would simply back his vehicle up and proceed to his next point of interest, giving the cleanup staff an opportunity to earn their wages.

When Germaine did catch up to Willie, his basket was full. And on top of the pile of goods sat charcoal and lighter fluid, ready to put Willie's culinary skills to the test. "I'm grilling tonight," he said. "Steaks."

Visions of their home burning to the ground and everything dear to her engulfed in flames filled Germaine's head. *Grilling indeed.*

"Willie, we're putting those back."

He refused.

"Willie?"

"No, we need them so I can make dinner for us tonight on my Weber," he said, as if completely oblivious to the limitations his illness had placed on him.

Now, Germaine had a new kind of blaze to extinguish: Willie's ill-thought-out way of taking care of things. But it wasn't in her heart to impose constant restrictions—his disease had already done that. Maintaining her husband's dignity was uppermost in Germaine's mind. All she could do was come down with firmness when she absolutely had to for his safety.

"Willie, if you don't put those back, I'm leaving you here at the store."

The charcoal and lighter fluid were out of his basket in seconds.

Wrong Joe, Right Joe

The adult day care center offered a program for patients with a wide variety of afflictions. While Helenn wanted to care for Joe at home, she knew she couldn't be his sole source of intellectual and social stimulation. After all, her husband had retired after a long profession that kept him in the limelight. His career, along with his robust involvement in philanthropic and charitable organizations, had frequently required his attendance at numerous and various social functions. With his gregarious personality, he savored his sociable lifestyle, so its diminishment was a loss for him. Joe's doctors could see it, too, and it was they who suggested Joe get together with other patients a few days a week for several hours.

On Joe's first day at the program, Helenn was happy to see her husband receive a nametag with a green dot. The attendant explained that green was code for "all systems go." This meant that Joe would be with a group of people who, like himself, were physically handicapped, but were normal cognitively. They could understand spoken language and follow directions, and they weren't at risk for running away. Joe's group would gather to play word games, discuss world events, and attend an art class to create drawings and paintings.

In the same room as the green-dot patients were those whose nametags bore yellow dots. These were folks who were fairly high functioning, but they required more caution. They might try to get out, for example, or they might tip over, or even throw, their coffee.

The red-dot day visitors were the ones to watch out for. Not only were they physically challenged, they were not aware enough to recognize the danger they might put themselves into.

It was the job of the receiving attendant to make sure each visitor went to the right group, and that everyone got safely into their caregivers' vehicles or the shuttle that would take them home at the end of the day.

Helenn and Joe were thrilled with the program. Helenn could still be her husband's primary caregiver, but now she would have time to run errands, take care of the home, and visit with friends. And Joe, much to his gladness, had a new social life.

One day while Helenn was at home, her friends John and Fay came by to visit. Topics of conversation flew back and forth between them like a heated badminton volley: job changes, neurological issues, caregiving. Suddenly, the doorbell rang. Helenn walked casually to the door, finishing her sentence before opening it. There, standing on the front step stood two men: the shuttle driver from the adult day center, and a stranger.

"Yes? Can I help you?" Helenn was confused.

The driver was equally confused. "We've brought your husband home, ma'am," he said.

Helenn looked past the other person as if he were invisible. "Where?" she asked.

The driver's eyes shifted to the side, as if to point out that this was her husband—without hurting her husband's feelings. "Right here." The stranger grinned.

"That's . . . not . . . my husband. But have a good day." Helenn moved to shut the door.

"Yes, I am your husband," said the man. "And I'd like to come in now."

By now, John and Fay were standing next to Helenn. "That's not Joe," John assured the driver.

"Yes, I am," said the man. His smile grew across his face as he stepped inside the door.

"Yes, he is," the driver insisted, pointing at the large, unambiguous letters on the red-dotted nametag: J-O-E.

As Helenn stared at the nametag, she suddenly realized what had happened. A quick phone call to the center solved the mystery of the errant Joe.

Attached to every red-dotted nametag was a sensor that would trip an alarm if its bearer wandered away. Somehow this Joe had removed his sensor, so when the driver came to pick up a man named Joe, red-dotted Joe had said, "Here I am. I'm Joe."

And off he went, undetected, through the doors and on his way to

Helenn's home.

"The wrong Joe is here," said Helenn calmly to the receptionist on the phone. "I'm sending him back to you. Please send the right Joe."

Hardly Injured

Family lore from Fred's youth wove itself into his and JoAnn's life in comical ways. In one such story, the childhood Fred had been merely an observer; his younger brother, George, had been the culprit. One day, Fred, George, and the boys' father were working in the family's gigantic garden. Suddenly George hurled something—surely nothing more menacing than a cucumber or a carrot green—but it whizzed by his father, missing him by centimeters.

"What are you trying to do, kill me?" shouted the eldest gardener.

"No, just injure you a little," was George's snappy comeback.

Well, Fred took that wisecrack right into his marriage. For years, if he did something, such as accidentally bump into JoAnn, she'd say, "What are you trying to do, kill me?"

"No, just injure you a little," he'd reply.

Or they'd tweak it to the situation. When JoAnn was irritated with her husband, for instance, she'd threaten him in the most benign way she could. "I'm going to kill you, Fred."

He'd laugh her off, of course. "No, just injure me a little."

As his illness progressed, Fred was no longer able to speak or read. Nevertheless, he loved his magazines and he loved sorting. So he spread his periodicals across the floor and placed them in various categories. All the same titles together. All cover pictures related in some way together in their own pile. Or all in alphabetical order. Thinking of new ways to organize his magazines kept him entertained—and mentally stimulated—for hours.

One day JoAnn took advantage of Fred's absorption in his journals to slip outside and water the garden. It was relaxing for her, and the rainbows that appeared in the gentle spray always tickled her. Rainbows in water. Peace in chaos. Hope in discouragement. Joy in trials. For JoAnn, it was almost a prayer.

Suddenly, the familiar sound of Fred's help signal broke her meditation. She had purchased a doorbell that sat on the table next to Fred so he could alert her with relatively little effort. Although this call didn't sound particularly frantic, she knew she needed to get to him as quickly as she could. So she untangled the hose, laid it on the grass, ran across the patio, stepped over the dog, darted through the patio door, and just as she fixed her eyes on her husband in an attempt to assess his situation, her feet flew out from under her. Fred had left one of his glossy magazines on the floor. Like a child on a Slip N Slide, but without the glee, she sailed across the floor, hit the ground—hard—and continued to careen right into the wall.

Fred laughed. Long after his voice had gone, those chortles were still there, ready to pounce on the whimsicalities he witnessed. But JoAnn was not amused. She grabbed a magazine and bopped him on the head.

"I'm going to kill you, Fred. I'm just going to kill you." Her voice was not kind. Her swat was not gentle.

Fred was stunned. He stopped laughing.

JoAnn felt horrible.

But then she saw that look in his eyes, the one that assured her everything was all right. The look that relieved the tension.

Without uttering a word, Fred told his wife, "No, just injure me a little."

Fudgsicles to the Rescue

The worst incident Annette can remember happened on New Year's Eve. Her husband, Mike, had been exhibiting compulsive behavior by standing in front of their decorative countertop in the living room—for twelve straight hours. Despite her best efforts to coax him into sitting down—including ice cream, her usual "carrot"— he was intent on standing.

It was clear Mike had a mission, but Annette didn't know what it was. He tried his best to communicate with her through all the means he knew: typing on his iPad, writing on newspapers and tissue boxes, scribbling on sheet after sheet of paper. But to Annette, it all looked like gibberish; she just couldn't understand what he was trying to say.

By late evening, Mike was on the verge of collapse. Agitated for lack of sleep, he was, to put it mildly, a handful. But still he would not sit down. Annette, now desperate, considered calling the paramedics, or even the police, but what would she tell them? *My husband is standing and won't sit down?* That hardly sounded like an emergency. She grew more anxious when she was unable to reach Mike's doctors or even his hospice caseworkers.

Twelve straight hours of standing. That couldn't be safe. And were they ever going to get to sleep? Nightmares of an overnight stand-up party were more than Annette could bear.

She finally called for an ambulance to take her husband to a nursing home.

Enter two burly EMTs, ready for the challenge. While they worked on calming Mike with an IV drip, Annette threw his clothes into a laundry basket and packed up his toiletries for his stay at the nursing home. But despite the sedation, Mike's manic energy continued to accelerate. Annette watched helplessly—and gratefully—as the EMTs escorted her husband down the front ramp while he bellowed like the Pharaoh crossing the Red Sea.

Then suddenly she remembered.

She ran to the freezer and grabbed the only tool she knew would work on Mike: a Fudgsicle. Racing to her husband's side, she plugged his mouth with the succulent chocolate pop. No more noise out of *him*.

The EMTs burst into laughter. "Well, we've never seen this before," one chuckled.

And off they went, leaving Annette to a quiet home, a place to rest, and a bed.

The twelve-hour standoff was over. She conked out within minutes.

Parkinson's Great Symphony

One of the hardest parts about having a neurodegenerative disease is that it's often misdiagnosed, at least in the beginning. It takes shrewd detective work—and some trial and error—to discern the source of a person's movement abnormalities, and those with the label "parkinsonism" or "atypical Parkinson's" are especially complex. Tremors, slow movement, impaired speech, and muscle stiffness may have a different cause than Parkinson's itself.

Phil's physician gave him the correct diagnosis, multiple system atrophy, but since MSA was such a rare disease, he suggested Phil tell people he had Parkinson's disease. That way, listeners would have a general idea of what Phil was going through, and he and Barb wouldn't have to spend a lot of time explaining all the symptoms and ramifications of MSA.

The doctor also recommended they go to the annual Parkinson's symposium near their home. His hope was that MSA would be mentioned there as a related disease, and the couple would gain more insight about Phil's condition. So far, Phil's parkinsonism was limited to a lack of balance. Fortunately, other symptoms they had heard about were not a concern, at least not yet.

During the morning sessions of the symposium, Phil and Barb listened to the ABCs—and XYZs—of Parkinson's disease until their brains were ready to burst. When lunch was finally announced, their relief was visible. The thrill of replacing words like "akinesia," "bradykinesia," and "cogwheel rigidity" with the simplicity of "asparagus," "bread," and "chicken" was a welcome thought.

The couple walked toward the huge conference center dining room, where the event planners had spared no adornment: linen-covered tables, colorful centerpieces, trees laden with twinkling lights bordering the room.

And hummingbirds. The pleasant buzzing was a regular ode to joy.

But looking around, expecting to see cages of birds for ambiance, Barb and Phil saw no birds at all, only people. People with Parkinson's disease. People whose trembling coffee cups and soup bowls—a symphony of hundreds—were clattering against their saucers, creating the avian sound effects.

And the royal blue carpeting and brilliant white tablecloths were covered with food. Beverages, salad, entrée makings, chunks of bread, desserts—every course was represented on the floor of the conference center dining room of the Parkinson's symposium.

Noise, Glorious Noise

Ear by ear, Mike lost his hearing. It was just one more hammering he would suffer in his decline, but he and his wife, Annette, reluctantly grew used to it, finding other ways to communicate: writing, drawing, lip-reading.

Charades.

But recent advances in cochlear implants would give Mike a chance to hear again. After his surgery, as the couple sat in the doctor's office, the sudden earsplitting ring of a cell phone pierced the air. At least that's how Mike heard it. He jerked his head toward the source of the sound, and his eyes lit up like a child's at the circus. It had been so long since he'd heard that glorious jingle.

Later that day, Mike opened a can of soda and nearly overflowed with merriment at the sound of fizzing carbon. His eyes moist with tears, the normally quiet, somewhat reserved engineer uttered a new mantra: "Oh, bubbles, bubbles, bubbles."

Pure joy.

But the biggest gift of Mike's restored hearing was, in fact, for Annette: she could finally turn down the TV.

Taming Mr. Handyman

ermaine was at her wit's end. Her lifetime of a handyman husband, Willie, kept forgetting he had limitations. Oh, she'd been grateful for his skills over the course of their married life; there wasn't a crack he couldn't patch, wire he couldn't hook up, or broken machine he couldn't mend, and his know-how had saved them thousands of dollars. But on this day she wasn't so sure how grateful she was.

"Willie, what is this?" she asked, trying to hide her sigh, her rolling eyes, her slumping shoulders. She pointed to the paint-covered duct tape over the door, then to the carpet where all his tools were spread out.

But she already knew what he was going to say.

"I fixed the hole in the door," he said, insinuating she was missing the obvious.

"Of course you did." Germaine ran her hand over the patch. *Another job for Angie's List,* she thought. The referral network of reputable home-repair specialists had been a lifesaver for her on many of Willie's post-diagnosis attempts to get his hands on much-needed repairs around the house. Sometimes she was lucky enough to catch him before he jammed the sander or electric drill into the surface of whatever he deemed needed fixing, but today she'd arrived too late.

Germaine glanced to her left. *Hmm.* "Willie, why is that table turned around?" She didn't really need to ask. He had run into it countless times with his wheelchair, and each time, he had, shall we say, "restored" it with Old English oil.

"Not worth fixing," he snorted. "So I just turned it around. Looks good as new, huh?"

At their family doctor's suggestion, the couple had obtained an electric wheelchair to use at home. What a disaster. Willie ran into furniture, doors, and cabinets right and left, and one day he tried turning around in a space that was too small, tearing a large hole in the wall. Willie didn't see this as a problem—because he could fix anything, remember?

Before long, Willie came up with the idea to invest in a shed so he could store his tools there. "Willie, we can't do that," Germaine said. "You know as well as I do that the neighborhood covenants won't allow it."

Willie grunted. "A handyman's gotta have a shed," he insisted, as he arranged his unhoused tools on the kitchen counter, first one way, then another.

"Let's just put them in the garage, why don't we?" said his wife.

He grunted again. "My garage is my garage. We need a shed for the tools."

Germaine sighed.

One day, Willie's granddaughter came to take him shopping. It was to be a lovely grandfather-granddaughter date, with Willie treating her to lunch afterward. But after several hours of shopping—and no lunch—a hungry and flustered granddaughter dropped Willie off at home. No explanation. No sentimental details about their special outing. She just let him in, turned around, and shut the door behind her. Germaine stifled a chuckle. *Welcome to my world*, she thought.

Three weeks later, the blare of the telephone broke the early morning silence. It was someone at Lowe's, wondering when they could deliver the shed.

"WILLIE!" Germaine did not disguise her displeasure. "Why did Lowe's just call about a shed?"

"We need a shed," he said matter-of-factly, keeping his eyes glued to a magazine he wasn't reading.

"So this is what you did when you took your granddaughter on a date? I'm going to call them back and cancel your order." Germaine knew she was in for a battle.

"No. We need a shed."

Several hours passed, and Willie wouldn't budge. Finally, Germaine had little choice but to resort to threats.

"Willie, which one of your children do you want to go live with? Because if I see a shed in that backyard, you and your clothes are going out the front door."

The handyman did not get his shed.

But Willie's reputation as a fix-it man followed him to the care center. One brisk day, Germaine walked into the dining hall, thinking she might help Willie clean up after his meal then take him back to his room. The large dining area was eerily silent, a surprising contrast to the normal hum of sweeping spoons, slurping, slopping, and voices of residents who were glad to be out of their lonely rooms for a spell. Then Germaine spotted four staff members at the back of the room, all staring down at the floor, so she walked over to see what was going on. There was Willie, down on his hands and knees, fixing a table. Seems he'd noticed that some of the tables were unstable, and had fashioned spacers out of cardboard to place under each leg.

Of every table.

In the entire dining hall.

Willie never looked up, so focused was he on his mission. Wobbly tables were his nemesis.

Feigning a tinge of exasperation, Germaine sat down to join the staff as they waited patiently for Willie to finish his work. Secretly, her heart swelled with pride toward her skilled husband.

She knew all too well that the man could not be tamed.

Close Encounters Where the Deer and the Antelope Play

When Phil received the diagnosis of a neurodegenerative disease, the doctor was clear that a decline was inevitable, but that they could and should live normally for as long as possible. Phil and his wife, Barb, took that advice and adjusted to the limitations as they came. But sometimes a situation would arise without warning, and they would barely catch it in time.

Barb's realization that Phil shouldn't be driving was one of those.

Still free of any discouraging challenges thus far, the two were on one of their frequent cross-country road trips, and Barb was at the wheel. It had been a particularly scenic drive as they headed west, with idyllic lakes and fir-lined hillsides dotted with deer and antelope, and the skies were not cloudy all day. They wanted it to last forever.

But the sun was beginning to dip below the horizon, and it was time to stop for the night. The problem was that each hotel they passed seemed worse than the last, so the couple decided to keep driving until something better popped up.

Barb waited until the traffic had dwindled down to almost nothing before handing over the driving to Phil. While Phil kept his eyes on the road, Barb kept hers peeled for a decent hotel, hoping one would turn up soon. So far, nothing filled the clearing between trees except a gas station or two, but she kept looking—to the right, then to the left, then to the right again.

Suddenly she let out a scream.

"Phil, watch out!"

Right next to the car, contrasting against the grayish sky, but clearly blocked by Phil's lack of peripheral vision, was an enormous moose.

"Oh," said Phil, unfazed. "I didn't see it."

"Oh," said Barb, her voice a tad shaky. "I see a hotel up ahead. Why don't we pull off?"

Who cares where we stay, anyway? she conceded, wiping her brow.

The Noble Cause of Preserving Dignity

D ignity was always in the forefront of Annette's mind while caring for Mike during his illness. But Mike, who had always been a rugged and independent guy, often bucked the doting he needed from his wife as his decline continued. Annette occasionally tried to bribe him to muster more cooperation.

"Actually, I think I bullied him at times," she playfully admits. But no matter how exasperating the situation, she made sure he always retained the option to say no.

As the most significant member of his care team, Annette took on Mike's daily shower routine. But she faced challenges as she tried to guide him onto his seat in the stall. No matter how many helper bars she installed in the shower, the naked truth was that soap is slippery. Very slippery. It was a thud waiting to happen every time.

So she came up with a solution.

"It was a little unconventional," she says. "But what the hell. I needed to shower too." So she would just settle him onto his chair in the large shower area—and jump in with him.

To show him he wasn't alone in needing daily care.

To preserve his dignity.

Annette, of course, took her responsibility seriously, and always made sure Mike got clean. But one time she let him experiment with the conditioner she used. He decided he liked it, and soon demanded she use it on him every day—and massage it in thoroughly, will you please, don't just dump it on my head.

To preserve his dignity, she complied.

Mike could hold a sponge and dab her here and there, which she was glad to let him do. It saved her a little time and energy. And when he changed his "target," she didn't object. Mike was a guy, and a guy he would be until the end.

Suffice it to say, Annette never had to wash her own chest. After all, she had to preserve his dignity.

Listen for the Thud and Watch for the Thug

When caregivers of patients with progressive supranuclear palsy get together to compare stories, one common thread of wisdom always comes up: just listen for the thud. Because experienced caregivers know two things: The first is that being right next to your patient at all moments is a physical impossibility.

The second is that it's a *given* they'll fall. So just listen for the thud.

Helenn heard the thud that day a few short minutes after Joe had shuffled down the hallway toward the bathroom. Practically a paramedic herself by now, she raced to his side and attempted to pick him up. He wouldn't budge. And because his legs were now rigid from the ravages of PSP, Joe could no longer do much to help the rescue efforts he and Helenn had perfected together.

"I need your cell phone, Joe." When Joe was finally able to extract his arm from the pretzel his body had become, Helenn gently removed the phone that was attached to his wrist. Dead. *Oh gosh, I have to be better about keeping the batteries charged,* she admonished herself. Seeing her husband sprawled helplessly on the floor, she grimaced.

Helenn sprinted to the other room to retrieve her own cell phone, which she normally kept in a black holder attached to her ankle where it wouldn't get lost or jarred. *Helenn, Helenn, Helenn,* she silently chided, *this is why you have a phone. You need to be more heedful about keeping it with you.* She dialed 911.

"Hello? This isn't a huge emergency, but my husband has fallen, and I can't lift him up off the floor." Helenn's phone calls to the fire department were becoming routine.

"And please don't use a siren," she pleaded as always. "Take your time. We're fine till you get here, and the door will be unlocked as usual."

217

She put her phone back in her ankle holder where it belonged.

Within minutes, four paramedics marched through the door and took their posts. Two righted Joe and carried him to his easy chair while a third took down information from soft-spoken Helenn.

The fourth was just making sure the operation ran smoothly. But Helenn noticed that his eyes kept darting from her to each of his colleagues, and back to her—over and over—as he fired off his questions.

Then he addressed Joe directly. "Do you need us to stay, sir?" Eyes flashed back to Helenn.

"Want us to call a friend or family member . . . or *someone* . . . for you?" Eyes flitted from Joe to Helenn, to fellow paramedics, back to Helenn.

"Are you sure you're going to be okay?" He tilted his head toward Helenn, as if some kind of code between himself and Joe.

What odd behavior, Helenn told herself. She walked the paramedics to the door.

Just then her cell phone rang. All eyes dropped to Helenn's ankle. All ears listened as she answered her call.

The hypervigilant paramedic finally seemed to relax. He exhaled loudly. "Whew. It's not an ankle monitor. Thank God."

Helenn looked confused.

The paramedic laughed. "I was afraid I was leaving Joe with someone who was under house arrest."

Healing from Loss

Sonja's loss was so great that she truly believed her life was over after Ken died. She was sure there would never be anything to look forward to again. For fifteen months, she stayed home, slept a lot, and kept a low profile. Her only outside activity was attending the caregivers' support group, hoping she could at least be of help to someone else.

But within a year, she had left the group. Sonja just preferred being in the comforting cocoon of her house.

Her daughter tried to get her interested in something—anything—but Sonja was content to stay at home. "The problem is," she says, "the more you stay at home, the more satisfied you become to just stay there."

Then one day a friend invited Sonja to a dance that night. She said no at first, then reluctantly acquiesced, but she literally had to drag herself out of the house.

Once the two friends stepped into the dance hall that evening, the lively music, ambient lights, and flurry of energetic dancers in their bright colors emanated contagious joy, and Sonja couldn't help but join in. Not only did she dance, she met new people and talked throughout the entire night.

Something in Sonja shifted for the first time in over a year. Her dance movements released endorphins, the conversations uplifted her, and she surprised herself when she left the dance in high spirits.

But once she got home, an unexpected feeling descended on her: she felt guilty that she had enjoyed the dance. She wept that night, sad that Ken hadn't been there to dance with her.

Perhaps Ken visited her that night, because a cliché she'd heard many times suddenly popped into her mind: life is for the living.

The truth was, she was alive—and she loved dancing. To have

nothing to look forward to would be a sad life indeed. Sonja pictured Ken encouraging her to be happy, to love life, to dance.

Sonja looked at the wedding photo that graced their living room. It gave her an urgency to share with other caregivers the wisdom she gained from the darkness following Ken's death: "Go through the cycles of grief, but make yourself get out and discover that there *is* life after you've lost your loved one. Allow it to happen."

She took a breath. "Never for a minute will I forget the life and love Ken and I shared for twenty-eight years. His love was the greatest gift of my life. But with his blessing, I believe, I can have fun now, and I look forward to every day. I never thought I would say this, but I'm truly happy again."

APPENDIX

DEFINITIONS OF TERMS

While an in-depth medical analysis of the conditions mentioned in these stories is beyond the scope of this book, a brief description of what caregivers of patients with degenerative neurological diseases face is relevant.

The diseases mentioned in this tome—PSP, MSA, CBD, and Lewy body disease—fall into the category of parkinsonism. They have no known cause, treatment, or cure.

Parkinsonism refers to a variety of pathologic conditions that have symptoms similar to those of Parkinson's disease: slow movement, tremors, stiffness, problems with balance, and trouble talking, sleeping, chewing, and swallowing. Because progressive supranuclear palsy (PSP), multiple system atrophy (MSA), and corticobasal degeneration (CBD) resemble Parkinson's disease, they are often misdiagnosed as Parkinson's, at least initially. The difficulty lies in the overlapping symptoms of the two, even though the pathology is different. Parkinson's disease, a movement disorder that develops when nerve cells in the brain fail to produce adequate amounts of the brain chemical dopamine, responds to dopamine-replacement therapy, such as Sinemet; parkinsonism does not. Often the determining factor in making a correct diagnosis is the response of the patient to dopamine-replacement therapy.

Progressive supranuclear palsy. Described as a disorder distinct from Parkinson's disease, **PSP** is a rare neurodegenerative brain disorder. A classic symptom, the inability to aim the eyes properly, is embedded in the disorder's long name: it begins gradually and gets progressively worse ("progressive"), causes weakness ("palsy"), by damaging parts of the brain above pea-sized structures called nuclei ("supranuclear") that control eye movements. Symptoms include:

- loss of balance
- impaired gait
- changes in personality such as increased irritability or diminished interest in pleasurable activities
- weak eye movement, especially in the downward direction
- trouble with movement of the mouth, tongue, and throat, resulting in slurred speech and difficulty swallowing
- difficulty finding expression to reflect the intelligence that is "locked inside"

Multiple system atrophy. MSA is a rare progressive disorder of the central and sympathetic nervous systems. Symptoms are related to the loss of nerve cells in several areas of the brain and spinal cord. They may include:

- lack of balance and coordination
- slow movement and stiff muscles
- progressive loss of motor skills
- slurred speech
- abnormal breathing and difficulty swallowing
- inability to sweat
- loss of bladder control
- irregular heart rate
- orthostatic hypotension, an excessive drop in blood pressure when the patient stands up, which causes dizziness or momentary blackouts

Corticobasal degeneration (CBD) is a rare neurodegenerative brain disease that affects nerve cells that control walking, balance, mobility, vision, speech, and swallowing. Symptoms come on asymmetrically, occurring on one side of the body first, then gradually moving to the other side, and include:

- Stiffness, shakiness, jerkiness, slowness, and clumsiness in either the upper or lower extremities

- Impaired speech generation and articulation
- Difficulty controlling the muscles of the face and mouth
- Walking and balance difficulty
- Memory or behavior problems

Lewy body disease, one of the most common causes of dementia, occurs when abnormal structures called Lewy bodies build up in areas of the brain. Symptoms include:

- Problems with movement and posture
- Muscle stiffness
- Changes in alertness and attention
- Hallucinations
- Confusion
- Loss of memory

TIPS FOR CAREGIVERS

Following is a list of helpful suggestions compiled by support group members in hopes of making the journey easier for their fellow caregivers. Special acknowledgement to Pat Hagan and John Jenkins for their leadership in compiling this brief directory in March 2014.

Please be advised that this is not a compendium of medical advice, but rather tidbits of experience provided by caregivers for caregivers. **Caregivers should never attempt to treat their patients before consulting a medical professional.**

BALANCE ISSUES

- Install **grab bars and poles** wherever the patient walks.
- Use a **gait belt**, a belt that the caregiver can grab onto in order to prevent the patient from falling. It is used to transfer the patient from one position or location to another. (**www.youtube.com/ watch/5Dr2NCd_YNg**)
- Provide a cane or walker. The **U-Step Walker**, paid for by Medicare, is weighted, which helps keep the patient upright. (**www.ustep.com/walker.htm**)
- To prevent injuries from falls, common safety accessories sold at sporting goods stores, such as bicycle helmets, wrist guards, elbow guards, and hip padding, are effective.

BATHROOM

- Raise the toilet seat so the patient doesn't lose balance when bending to sit. This also makes it easier for the caregiver to assist the patient in sitting and standing.

- Install **security poles** for the patient to hold onto while sitting down and getting up. Some poles have curved grab bars on them, such as the **HealthCraft Super Pole**, and others do not. Security poles can be placed anywhere the patient walks throughout the house. (**www.stander.com**)

BEDRAIL

In addition to keeping the patient from sliding off the mattress, a bedrail also gives the patient something to grab onto when getting out of bed.

BEDRIDDEN

When the time comes to set up a hospital bed in the home, it's important to get a totally electric one. The alternative is to hand-crank the head of the bed up and down—often many times throughout the day.

BEDSORES (also called ulcer sores or pressure sores)

- Bedridden patients are at risk for developing pressure sores, which are injuries to the skin and underlying tissue resulting from prolonged pressure against a surface. For this reason, the patient needs to be turned frequently.
- Special pressure relief mattresses, which help prevent bedsores, are provided by hospice along with the hospital bed.

BLADDER PROBLEMS

- Absorbent underpants, available from **www.tranquilityproducts.com**, keep urine away from the patient's skin and neutralize odor.
- Catheters can cause irritation, so many caregivers avoid using them until absolutely needed. But once that time comes, many

caregivers have found that catheterization makes it much easier to care for the patient.

- Prescription Detrol or Enablex can diminish the sense of urgency.

BOWEL PROBLEMS

- Most importantly, give plenty of fluids to avoid dehydration.
- Use generous amounts of fiber in the patient's diet, such as All-Bran cereal, vegetables, fruits, and Prunelax.
- Psyllium and MiraLAX are also helpful. Start with small doses and add more as necessary.
- Some caregivers put a tablespoon of oil in or on the patient's food, then serve a helping of pureed prunes.
- Promote regularity by helping the patient to the toilet at the same time every day.
- For protection, patients seem to prefer pull-on disposable adult underpants rather than adult diapers.
- Using shaving cream to clean bowel mishaps is gentle on the patient's skin and, when used in tandem with dry wipes, works better than Wet Ones flushable wipes alone.
- Some caregivers have found success using probiotics for regularity.

BRAIN BANK

Patients with rare neurodegenerative diseases might consider making arrangements in advance to donate brain tissue to the **Mayo Clinic Brain Bank** in Jacksonville, Florida. The family will receive confirmation of their loved one's actual disease. A brochure and the necessary forms are available to download and print at **www.curepsp.org**.

"BUSINESS CARDS"

Doctors, nurses, friends, relatives, and home health caregivers may all appreciate a "business card," which can be printed with an explanation of the patient's illness. This is especially helpful in the case of relatively unknown diseases such as PSP and MSA, and where the patient's movements can be easily misinterpreted.

COMMUNICATION

- If the patient is no longer able to speak, establish a set of hand signals. Ask yes-no questions that can be answered with one finger up for yes, two up for no.
- Depending on the disease and the patient's stage, electronic communication devices can be helpful.
- Speech therapy can be helpful for some.
- **The Tremble Clefs Program** is a nationwide therapeutic singing program for people with Parkinson's disease and parkinsonism, and their caregivers. The program, available through the American Parkinson Disease Association, establishes singing groups in which individuals address voice and communication problems through breathing, stretching and posture activities, vocal exercise, rhythm and movement, and a strong social support system.

COUGHING AND DROOLING

- These are sometimes caused by excess saliva, gastric reflux, or lung infection.
- Caregivers may need to suction extra saliva. Suction machines are provided by home health care and hospice.
- Many caregivers report success with Botox injections to control excess saliva, but some patients have experienced adverse reactions.

DYING

Some caregivers recommend this hour-long YouTube video, conducted by a hospice nurse: **www.youtube.com/watch/PPx-qpos57g**.

EATING

- When the patient can no longer feed himself, use plastic or cloth "bibs," such as those found at **www.wrightstuff.biz**.
- Use Velcro to fasten cloth bibs.
- Slanted plates and bowls with lips, combination forks and spoons, and Nosey Cups, which have a special cutout that helps maintain proper head and neck positioning when swallowing, are all valuable mealtime tools.
- When the patient has trouble swallowing, puree his food. **The Magic Bullet** blender serves this purpose well (**www. buythebullet.com**). Also see **Thickeners** and **Tube Feeding**.

EYES, DOUBLE VISION

Glasses with prisms may help, at least for a while.

EYES, WATERING

Using eye drops or eye gel three to four times a day can help watering eyes. Caregivers suggest non-preservative types like Systane eye drops and Systane eye ointment or gel. If the cells in the eyes die, it can be painful, so see an ophthalmologist regularly.

HOME HEALTH CARE

Speech therapy, physical therapy, and occupational therapy can all be helpful. Some home healthcare agencies are good, some are not. Follow the advice of doctors, nurses, and other experienced caregivers.

HOSPICE

When modern medicine cannot offer a cure, many families choose hospice care, whether in the patient's home or in a hospice facility. A care team will provide:

- management of pain and other symptoms
- emotional and spiritual support
- medications, medical supplies, and medical equipment
- family support
- short-term inpatient care as respite for the family when pain and other symptoms become too difficult to manage at home

Many areas have more than one hospice. Comprehensive information about hospice, including where to find one in your area, can be found at **www.hospicenet.org**. Also see **Palliative Care.**

INABILITY TO WALK OR STAND

- A lift chair, a motorized seat that lifts the patient to a standing position, is available through medical supply stores.
- Caregivers report the **Invacare Reliant 350 Stand-Up Lift** to be extremely helpful. Used chairs can be found online at less cost, or purchased from a caregiver whose loved one has passed.
- A video showing how to use the Invacare is available at **www. youtube.com/watch/pTkvbyTvhwg**.

LONG-TERM CARE INSURANCE

Many useful items, equipment, and services are covered by Medicare or hospice, but for those that are not, long-term care insurance can be a good solution.

MEDICAL ALARM SYSTEMS

- Many of these devices contact a central office for help.
- An alternative, the **Freedom Alert**, is available for a one-time purchase fee of about $300. Pressing a button on the device will dial the phone number of your choice, or 911. Learn more at **www.freedomalert-911.com**.

PAIN

Some patients have found prescription Lidoderm patches helpful for neck or back pain.

PALLIATIVE CARE

If your patient is not ready for hospice, a better choice might be palliative care—specialized medical attention that focuses on providing patients relief from the symptoms, pain, and stress of a serious illness. It is appropriate at any stage of a life-threatening disease and can be provided along with curative treatment. Most hospices can arrange for palliative care.

PHYSICIANS

- Families of patients with Parkinson's disease or parkinsonisms, such as PSP or MSA, stress the importance of seeing a **movement disorder specialist** in addition to retaining a relationship with their primary care physician or internist.
- For any life-threatening illness, the right specialist is essential. However, for rare diseases, it isn't always easy to figure out what the appropriate specialist is.

READING

- The **Merlin LCD by Enhanced Vision** is a machine that

magnifies the printed word for those who have difficulty reading, and displays it on a built-in LCD monitor, which resembles a computer.

- The Braille Institute has free audio books and magazines on tape that can be shipped to the patient postage-free or downloaded from the internet. The Braille Institute also offers free machines to play the material.
- Books on tape and CD are always available at public libraries.

SLEEP PROBLEMS

Some patients have benefited from using Benadryl plus three milligrams of melatonin. Of course, consult a physician before trying any sleep remedies.

STAIR LIFT

A stair lift is a moving chair, usually installed along the length of a staircase, that carries a patient from one level of the house to the next. **Bruno** and **Pacific Mobility** are brands that many caregivers find reliable.

TELEPHONES

- A cell phone is helpful for communicating when the caregiver is away from home. Be sure the caregiver's phone number is on speed dial.
- A phone wristwatch, the **Galaxy Gear**, is another handy communication device available from **Samsung**.
- Some caregivers attach cell phone holders to their patient's ankles.

THICKENERS

- When thin liquids cause a patient to cough, gag, or even choke, thickeners can be added.

- **Thick-It** is a brand of powder additive available at pharmacies and sometimes provided by hospice.
- **SimplyThick**, a liquid that comes in premeasured packets, is preferred by some because it has no taste.
- **Hormel Thick & Easy** is another thickening product recommended by some caregivers.

TRANSPORTATION

- Fold-up wheelchairs are available for moving the patient to and from the car.
- For getting in and out of the car, the **Handy Bar** is a useful tool and works on all makes and models. Available on **www. amazon.com.**
- The **CarCaddie** is a nylon strap with a plastic handle that attaches to a car door frame. Note that it doesn't work on frameless windows.
- Many cities and towns have free or low-cost shuttles for senior citizens, with accommodations for those with physical limitations.

TUBE FEEDING

For a patient who frequently chokes on her food or who can no longer eat for other reasons, tube feeding can prolong her life. The patient's quality of life and her desire to prolong that level of quality will determine the appropriateness of using a feeding tube.

URINARY TRACT INFECTION (UTI)

UTIs can become a big problem, especially with an indwelling catheter. Suprapubic catheters are a common solution.

WHAT IS HELPFUL, WHAT IS NOT

Caregivers often find themselves in a quagmire. Tending to the needs of loved ones with life-threatening or terminal illnesses makes caregivers both givers and receivers of assistance; they pour themselves into watching over their dear ones at the same time that they accept help from well-meaning friends and family. But both roles can put them in difficult positions. By and large, when compassionate friends rush to the sides of caregivers, showering them with acts of kindness and words of encouragement, the help is appreciated. But at times it may not be.

The caregivers in this book offer these insights about what helps and what does not. It's important to recognize that each individual and each family is in a different situation. Some gestures may be helpful for one family and not for another, so consider these general guidelines.

Helpful

- Send mail, with no expectation of receiving a response. Short or long cards, letters, and emails brighten a patient's—and a caregiver's—day. The patient and caregiver can read the sweet, funny, and encouraging words when they're up to it, and reread when they need a lift. In that way, mail is a gift that's ongoing.
- Offer to be the lead messenger. It's hard for a patient's family to be inundated with phone calls. But those interested in helping can find out the status of the patient with a quick email or phone call to a trusted person assigned by the patient's caregiver. In that role, the lead messenger can coordinate visits and phone calls, meals, and other acts of kindness.
- Be specific about offers of help. You would bend yourself into a pretzel to be of help, of course. The best way to make that known is to let the caregiver know exactly what you would like

to do and when. "I'm making roasted chicken tonight, and I'll bring it over at six unless I hear otherwise," or "I'll pick up the children for soccer practice at four o'clock each Tuesday and Thursday, unless you tell me not to," are welcome offers.

- Caregivers have especially appreciated these gifts: dinners that are sensitive to the family's dietary needs—and served in disposable dishes that don't need to be returned; healthy snack foods; videos, magazines, puzzles, and books that are easy reading; a jump rope, stretch tubing, small trampoline, or other space-saving equipment that encourages exercise for the caregiver.
- Be sensitive to differing religious traditions. People are at different milestones on the spiritual path at any given time, and moments of misfortune evoke varying responses in the afflicted and in the caregiver. Trials may cause a deepening in faith, but they may just as likely invoke feelings of abandonment by their God. The journey belongs to that person in a profound and personal way. Some caregivers have reported their discomfort when a group surrounds them in fervent prayer. Without a doubt, pray for the patient and caregiver in the silence of your heart, but only out loud if they request it or if you know it would be comforting to them because of your previous understanding of their faith life.
- Give long, hard, frequent hugs—with no words.

Not helpful

- "Call me if you need anything." This casts the caregiver into the role of beggar, a most vulnerable place to be.
- "Everything happens for a reason." This is hard for anyone to hear in the face of trial or tragedy. To the ears of the receiver, it sounds like the speaker is making light of their horrendous challenge. As one caregiver noted, "People try to create a narrative that makes sense to them. But it's theirs, not mine."
- Even comments such as "I wish I could take this challenge away

from you" can cause a pang in the listener. When caregivers choose to take care of their dear ones, they would rather hear encouragement for their choice.

- Being hurt. The patient and the caregiver are both immersed in an immensely stressful situation and may not respond as you would like. Don't take anything personally.

A word to caregivers on the receiving end of helpful gestures.

People who approach you are trying to help. They may make mistakes, they may say things that are irrelevant, seemingly insensitive, even hurtful. But do your best to accept the goodwill with which their efforts are offered. No one really knows what the other needs until he or she has been in that situation.

Acknowledgements

I wish to recognize those who made this book a reality.

Timothy Pike (www.dreamplaywrite.com) for your invaluable editing. Your mastery of the written word, and your suggestions, always gentle and respectful, made my manuscript the best it could be.

Betsy Pike and **Molly Pike**, your proofreading was superb, your observations about inconsistencies, impressive.

George McCann, MD, for helping me understand the science behind these devastating diseases and for your guidance in using medical terminology accurately, I thank you.

Denny Dressman, I appreciate your eye for detail, your encouragement, and your mentorship.

Caterine de Virgilio, even in casual conversation, your words sparkle. Thank you for your input and your help tweaking my words till I got it right.

Lynne Knickerbocker, you've inspired me your whole life with your love and wisdom. Now you inspire me on what you call your "road to Calvary."

Anne O'Konski (www.aokstudios.com) for your artistic brilliance and your help in turning our rough ideas into a beautiful cover.

The members of the Denver, Colorado, **PSP/MSA support group,** for generously sharing your stories and inspiring me to no end with your beautiful testaments to the power of love.

www.ingramcontent.com/pod-product-compliance
Lightning Source LLC
Chambersburg PA
CBHW021616270326
41931CB00008B/731